Avicenna On Healthy Living

Exercising, Ma... ...g,
Drinking, Slee... ...ue

...

Laleh Bakhtiar

From Translations by
O. Cameron Gruner and Mazar H. Shah
Correlated with the Arabic by Jay R. Crook
with Notes by O. Cameron Gruner

Great Books of the Islamic World, Inc.

Printed in the United States of America.

Library of Congress Cataloging-in-Publication Data

Ibn Sina, Abu Ali al-Husayn ibn Abd Allah
The Canon of Medicine (al-Qanun fi'l tibb)
Lecture 16 - Exercises for the Physically Mature
1. Islam. 2. Medicine. I. Title

ISBN 10 (Book): 1-56744-793-7
ISBN 13 (Book): 978-1-56744-793-4
ISBN 10 (eBook): 1-56744-794-5
ISBN 13 (eBook): 978-1-56744-794-1

Cover Design by Liaquat Ali
Cornerstones are Allah and Muhammad connected by Bismillah al-Rahman al-Rahim (In the Name of God, the Merciful, the Compassionate).

Design and layout by Abir Usman

Published by
Great Books of the Islamic World, Inc.

Distributed by
KAZI Publications, Inc.
3023 W. Belmont Avenue
Chicago IL 60618
Tel: 773-267-7001; FAX: 773-267-7002
email: info@kazi.org

Contents

Introduction by Laleh Bakhtiar

In the Name of God, the Merciful, the Compassionate

I. Biographical Sketch

The "Prince of Physicians," Abu Al Sina (Avicenna) (b. 370/980) was born in Afshana. By the age of ten he had learned the entire Quran as well as grammar and then began the study of logic and mathematics. Once these subjects were mastered, he studied physics, metaphysics and medicine. By the age of sixteen he had mastered all of the sciences of his day except metaphysics. While he had read Aristotle's Metaphysics over and over again and had even memorized it, he could not understand it until he read al-Farabi's commentary on it. Avicenna was then eighteen years old.

He was favored by the ruler of Bukhara because of his mastery of medicine, but when he was thirty-two, he was forced to migrate because of the political situation in his home town area. He migrated to Jurjan on the southeast coast of the Caspian Sea in an attempt to join the court of the well-known Qabus ibn Wushmgir. This never materialized as the ruler had died in 1013 during Avicenna's travels to Jurjan. Avicenna then retired to a village near Jurjan where he was to meet his disciple-to-be, al-Juzjani.

Al-Juzjani was devoted to Avicenna and was to write commentaries upon his works as well as to preserve copies of all of the master's writings. It was in Jurjan in 1012 that Avicenna wrote the beginning of his great medical text, *The Canon (al-Qanun)* on medicine. Avicenna remained in Jurjan for two or three years before moving to Rey in 405/1014 or 406/1015, a city near present day Tehran and from there to Hamadan in the northwest Iran. He became a minister in the Buyuid Court of Shams al-Dawlah as well as the court physician. Once again Avicenna was obliged to migrate because of the unstable political conditions in Hamadan so he moved to Isfahan where he enjoyed a fifteen year period of peace, writing many of his major works at that time.

Eventually, however, he was forced to migrate once again and moved back to Hamadan where he died in 428/1037.

II. Avicennian Corpus

One of the leading scholars on Avicenna and the editor of this series, Seyyed Hossein Nasr, has written the following:

> The writings of Avicenna, of which nearly 250 have survived, if we take all his short treatises and letters into account, range over nearly every subject known to the medieval world. These works are mostly in Arabic, but occasionally in Persian, as for example, the *Danish namah-i ala* (The Book of Science Dedicated to Ala al-Dawlah), which is the first philosophic work in modern Persian. Avicenna's Arabic style in his earlier works is rather difficult and uneven; and it was only during his long sojourn in Isfahan-when under the criticism of certain literary experts, he began to study Arabic literature intensely-that his style became polished and perfected. The works written later in life, especially the *Isharat wa'l tanbihat*, testify to this change.
>
> Aviennna's philosophical works include his Peripatetic masterpiece *al-Shifa* (The Book of the Remedy), the Latin *Sufficientia*, which is the longest encyclopedia of knowledge ever written by one man, his Najat (The Book of Deliverance), which is a summary of the *Shifa, Uyun al-hikmah* (Fountains of Wisdom), and his last and perhaps greatest masterpiece *Isharat wa 'l-tanbihat* (The Book of Directives and remarks). In addition he wrote a large number of treatises on logic, psychology, cosmology, and metaphysics. There are also the "esoteric" works pertaining to his "Oriental Philosophy" of which the *Risalah fi'l ishq* (Treatise on Love), the Trilogy *Hayy ibn Yaqan* (The Living Son of the Awake), *Risalat al-Tair* (Treatise of the Bird) and Salaman wa Absal, the last three chapters of the *Isharat*, and *Mantiq al-mashriqiyin* (The Logic of the Orientals), which is a part of a larger work now lost, are the most important.
>
> In the sciences, also, Avicenna composed many small treatises dealing with particular problems in physics, meteorology, and so on, as well as sections contained in the larger compendia, especially the *Shifa*, in which is found the most complete exposition of his views on zoology, botany, and geology, as well as psychology, which in Peripatetic philosophy—and contrary to the view of the later schools like the *Ishraqiyyun* is considered as a branch of physics or natural philosophy. As for medicine, Avicenna composed the famous *Qanun*, or *Canon*, which is perhaps the most influential single work in the history of medicine and is still taught in the East today, the *Urjuzah fi'l-tibb* (Poem on Medicine), containing the principles of Islamic medicine in rhyming verses easy to memorize, and a large number of treatises in both Arabic and Persian on various diseases and drugs.
>
> In addition to his philosophical and scientific works, Avicenna wrote several poems in Arabic and Persian of which *Qasidat al-ainiyah* (Ode on the Soul) is deservedly the most famous. Moreover, he wrote several religious works which include not only treatises on particular religious subjects, such as the meaning of fate and free will, but also commentaries upon several chapters of the Quran.

This latter category is particularly important because it was primarily in these commentaries that Avicenna sought to harmonize reason and revelation along lines already begun by *al-Kindi, al-Farabi* and the *Ikhwan al-safa*, continued after him by *Suhrawardi*, and finally brought to its fruition by *Mir Damad* and *Mulla Sadra*. These writings add an important dimension to the already multidimensional corpus of Avicenna's literary output and emphasize the richness of a collection of writings which range from observational and even experimental science to ontology, from mathematics to gnosis and metaphysics, and from logic to commentaries upon the Sacred Book.[1]

III. The Theory and Practice of Islamic Medicine

The traditional concept of medicine[2] differs profoundly from the view held in the modern world because in the traditional view, the spaces —meridians, channels—within the body and what flows through them are of more significance in causing illness than the shapes or organs, members themselves. That is, the emphasis is on that which flows through the channels as the "place" of the soul.

A clear parallel can be seen in traditional Islamic architecture where space is considered to be one of the most direct symbols of Being and it is primordial, all-pervading and, in Islamic cosmology, the locus of the Universal Soul. Space is also structured. Whether one is referring to the macrocosm or the microcosm, they each contain three divisions: body, soul and spirit.

> Traditional man tends towards a mode of comprehension which provides a metaphysical interpretation of life, an interpretation that precedes and goes beyond all external perception. This mode of comprehension, or initial interpretation, affects all of man's perceptions because it begins by situating him in the universe. Initially this interpretation determines his awareness of cosmic space as an externalization of the macrocosmic creation which is analogous to his own microcosmic self. This traditional Hermetic concept forms part of the world view incorporated into the Islamic perspective, a view in which the universe is composed of a macrocosm and microcosm, each containing three great divisions: the body (*jism*), the soul (*nafs*) and the spirit (*ruh*).[3]

Depending on one's perspective, one is either drawn from the body through the soul to the Divine Spirit in the external world or from the body inward through the soul to the Hidden Treasure or Divine Spirit within.

> Two interpretations of this concept arise which, although apparently different, are essentially the same. In the first, God as Manifest (*al-Zahir*), is the reality of universal externalization. From within the concentric circles of the macrocosm, there is an outward movement from the earth as

> corporeal manifestation through an all-pervading soul to the enveloping heavens, viewed as the seat of the Divine Spirit. In the second, complementary view of God as Hidden (*al-Batin*), there is an inward movement within the microcosm of man, beginning with his physical presence and moving towards his spiritual center, the Hidden Treasure. The two schemes correspond to each other, at the same time that one is the reverse of the other.[4]

In this structured space, the human being knows where he or she is. Direction is meaningful.

> It is only with reference to the heavens that the apparent indefiniteness of space can be given direction. In this way space acquires a qualitative aspect. The order of the spheres and the movements through the six directions of north, south, east, west, up and down constitute the primary coordinate system within which all creation is situated. All traditional sciences share this common frame of reference.[5]

The concept of place (*makan*) follows a meaningful direction or orientation. A sense of place consists of both a container (*jism*, body) and the contained (soul, spirit, breath).

> [The concept of place] does not have a tangible existence, but exists in the consciousness of the beholder who visually perceives physical boundaries while his intellect perceives [the soul] and spirit as 'contained,' defined within the boundaries.[6]

Within this structured, oriented concept of space as the place of the soul, all of creation contains both active and passive possibilities. The idea of time in motion arises from the active aspect of space while seen in its passive aspect, it is manifested in matter or form which is directly a product of this movement. This concept—that the soul (space) and not the body (shape) should lead in the healing art—is central to an understanding of traditional medicine.

> The esoteric theory of causation describes this motion as the movement of the soul towards the Divine Spirit through space. Thus the locus of time and form is space, which simultaneously manifests its active and passive aspects through motion.[7]

This perspective is the basis for traditional medicine which looks for the simultaneous movement systems which create a continuous flow based on number—three main faculties, three major organs, three souls, four elements, four humours, nine temperaments, and which interact in space, the place of the soul, with the organs, tissues, membranes, etc.

Finally, we come to the concept of rhythm in time which is best described in terms of traditional music based upon the poem with which Jalal al-Din Rum begins his masterful *Mathnawi*.

Hearken to this Reed forlorn,
Breathing, even since twas torn
From its rushy bed, a strain
Of impassioned love and pain.

The Secret of my song, though near,
None can see and none can hear.
Oh, for a friend to know the sign
And mingle all his soul with mine!

'Tis the flame of Love that fired me.
'Tis the wine of Love inspired me.
Wouldst thou learn how lovers bleed.
Hearken, hearken to the Reed![8]

The continuity and harmony of music is well appreciated and may serve to elucidate another aspect of the spiritual meaning of time-form continuity. The reed, in Jalal al-Din Rumi's poem, contains the bifold characteristics of place. Physically, the reed exhibits a *zahir* or external form which is passive to its hollow interior or *batin*, wherein lies the active spirit of the instrument. The music of the reed is symbolically seen as the externalization of an interior movement, just as musical tones work through wind instruments from the inside out. He who hears the music is aware of the inner space and the harmonious encounter of its motion with its outer shell. This interaction, in the traditional view, represents a spiritual synthesis which regards the reed's *zahir* as the body and its *batin* as the spirit, which, through the music of the soul, yearns to return to the reed bed from whence it was plucked, must as man yearns to return to the One from whom he was issued.[9]

The concept of motion associated with the creation of time and space is explored also by Ibn Arabi in his discourses on initial creation and the subsequent manifestations, viewed as the 'Breath of the Compassionate.' Here 'the universe is annihilated at every moment and re-created at the next without there being a temporal separation between the two phases. It returns back to the Divine Essence at every moment while in the phase of contraction and is re-manifested and externalized in that of expansion. . . Creation is renewed at every instant and its apparent 'horizontal' continuity is pierced by the 'Vertical Cause' which integrates every moment of existence into its transcendent Origin.'[10]

Because of the concentration of traditional Islamic medicine on what flows through the inner spaces, it becomes a dynamic system. That is, the whole is present and operative in each individual locus in which each individual locus knows, so to speak, its position in the whole, its relation to center. The dynamic qualities of the elements can be understood as manifestations of an orderly action of faculties (drives, energies, powers) within a given system. The elemental qualities of our body's system are part of a dynamic field and each elemental quality, as it presents itself, gives expression to the exact constellation of faculty that is present at the point at which the element is situated, a dynamic quality that permits the elemental qualities to become the conveyors of meaning; that makes temperaments out of the succession of elements.

Thus, we have introduced the traditional concepts of the soul and its place in space with the traditional components of space: structured (body, soul, spirit), oriented (six directions), sense of place (container/contained), positive space continuity (what flows through space creates shapes), time-form simultaneity (active as motion, passive as form), and rhythm in time (breath, pulse). Now let us turn to Avicenna. He begins *The Canon* with a definition of the science of medicine:

> Medicine (*tibb*) is the science by which we learn the various states of the human body in health and when not in health, and the means by which health is likely to be lost and, when lost, is likely to be restored back to health. In other words, it is the art whereby health is conserved and the art whereby it is restored after being lost.

Avicenna insists that the human body cannot be restored to health unless the causes of both health and disease are determined. In categorizing the causes, he uses Aristotle's system:

> Medicine deals with the states of health and disease in the human body. It is a truism of philosophy that a complete knowledge of a thing can only be obtained by elucidating its causes and antecedents, provided, of course, such causes exist. In medicine it is, therefore, necessary that causes of both health and disease should be determined.
>
> Sometimes these causes are obvious to the senses but at other times they may defy direct observation. In such circumstances, causes and antecedents have to be carefully inferred from the signs and symptoms of the disease. Hence, a description of the signs and symptoms of disease is also necessary for our purpose. It is a dictum of the exact sciences that knowledge of a thing is attained only through a knowledge of the causes and origins of the causes—assuming there to be causes and origins. Consequently our knowledge cannot be complete without an understanding both of symptoms and of the principles of being.

There are four causes—material, efficient, formal, and final. On the subject of health and disease, we have the following:

The Material Causes

The material (*maddi*) cause is the physical body which is the subject of health and disease. This may be immediate as the organs of body together with their vital energies and remote as the humours and remoter than these, the elements which are the basis both for structure and change (or dynamicity). Things which thus provide a basis (for health and disease) get so thoroughly altered and integrated that from an initial diversity there emerges a holistic unity with a specific structure (or the quantitative pattern of organization) and a specific type of temperament (the qualitative pattern).

The material cause, then is the physical body, as viewed from the traditional perspective. It consists of the organs, the breath, the humours and the elements. We begin with the elements as Avicenna does.

The Elements

The primary constituents of the human body in traditional medicine are called "the elements." They are the basic building blocks for the science of medicine.

The four elements—earth, air, fire, and water—are the simplest particles of all that is material. They are the simplest particles of our bodies. To each of them are joined two qualities. Earth is dry and cold; water, cold and moist; air, hot and moist; and fire is hot and dry. Earth is contrary to air and water to fire. Union is possible because water serves as a means between earth and air and air as a means between water and fire. The elements, like musical tones, possess an inclination not only to ascend and descend, but also to move in a circular direction. Each element is joined by one of its qualities to that which is below and by the other to that which is above it. Water to earth beneath by coldness and to air above by moisture; air to water beneath by moisture and to fire above by heat; fire to air beneath by heat and to earth toward which it declines by dryness; earth to water above by coldness and to fire which declines toward it by dryness. Two of the elemental qualities are active and two passive. Active are hot and cold. Passive are dry and wet. The resulting qualities, the ideal combination, is an equitable one.

Quality results from the opposing qualities of the elements, a mixture of hot, cold, wet and dry. Balance comes when the strength of primary qualities are equal to these qualities—an average of these qualities. In medicine, it does not depend upon exactly equal but "equitable," meaning that the quality and quantity of the elements are distributed in such a manner that the resulting pattern or equilibrium of the body as a whole or if its parts is the one most appropriate for that person.

When one quality predominates over the other, the body is not well suited to the needs of the soul. The proportion in which the elements are united with the body has an influence upon action. Slow and heavy moving signifies a predominance of cold and dryness (earth); fearfulness and sluggishness, of cold and wetness (water); cheerfulness, of heat and wetness (air); and sharp, angry violence, of heat and dryness (fire).

All physical forms consist of elemental qualities prefigured in the physical process. If something changes in the element, something must have changed in the physical process. The two stand to each other in the strict relationship of cause and effect.

As phenomena of the external world and, in traditional medicine, the inner world, consist of the elements and their qualities, as well. Different elemental qualities are always based on the different properties of the elements (higher, lower, lighter, heavier, colder, hotter, etc.). The distinguishing characteristic of the elements is that they differ like two colors, red and green, and like two shades of a single color, light and dark blue or like shapes rough and square. The property is a characteristic of such a nature that it both distinguishes different elements from one another and at the same time orders them in definite ways.

The dynamic quality of the elements is that they have direction. The elements point one to another—attract and are attracted—and are therefore directional forces. Elemental motion has its origin not in differences of properties but in differences of dynamic quality as conveyors of motion.

The Humours

The humours are the primary fluids of the body which move through inner space. These humours affect the function of the body and are themselves influenced by the states of motion and rest of the human being.

Food and drink are transformed into innate heat through the digestive process. The humours arise in the second stage of digestion in the liver. This process produces four humours which sustain and nourish the body and move through the channels or meridians: sanguineous (blood), serous (phlegm), bilious (choler, yellow bile) and atrabilious (melancholy, black bile) corresponding to air (hot and wet), water (cold and wet), fire (hot and dry) and earth (cold and dry). These are subject to variation in quantity and in degree of purity.

Illness results from either a quantitative or qualitative change of humour. In a "normal" state, the humours are assimilated by the organs and completely integrated into the tissues. In an "abnormal" state, due to improper digestion, the material is unsuitable for assimilation and therefore eliminated by the body. Surpluses may be eliminated by exercise, bathing, coition, purges and laxatives.

The sanguineous humour (blood), which is an equal temper, exceeds the others in proportion to quantity, is hot and moist, sweet and red. It imparts strength and color to the body and serves for the engendering of the drives. Located in the heart, it relates to Leo, Aries and Sagittarius in the Zodical constellations.

The serous humour or phlegm, next to blood in quantity, is watery, cold, moist and white. It moderates the strength, heat, and thickness of blood, nourishes the brain, and moistens and nourishes such part of the body as are concerned in motion. If blood fails, heat dissolves the serous humour into blood. Cancer, Pisces and Scorpio, as Zodiacal signs, relate to serous humour.

The bilious humour, least in quantity, is hot and dry, yellow or red and bitter. A part of it passes from the liver to the gallbladder and a part, flowing thence with other humours, moderates moisture and makes the blood subtle so that it may pass easily through straight ways. The bilious humour prevents the body from becoming heavy, sleepy and dull. It penetrates and opens passages and feeds members of the body in which the fiery element predominates. Zodiacal signs are Gemeni, Aquarius, and Libra.

The atrabilious humour is earthy and gross, thick, black and sour. A part of it passes to the spleen and a part remains with the blood. This humour feeds the bones, the spleen and other parts of the body which are gross or "melancholy" in nature. It tempers the two hot humours (sanguineous and bilious) and serves to stay and retain the floating spirits that arise from blood. The atrabilious humour thickens the blood and thus prevents it from flowing too freely through the veins and arteries. Within the Zodaic this humour is related to the three signs Tarus, Virgo, and Capricorn.

From the natural predominance of a humour in the human being spring definite characteristics of physique and conduct. Those dominated by the sanguinious humour are cheerful, courageous, kind and ingenious. Their blood, if subtle, makes the wit keen. As fatness increases, blood diminishes. The serous humour dominating is visible in people who are easily provoked, given to treachery and vehement in action; fierce in assailing but inconstant in sustaining the assault; inclined to envy, pride, prodigality and wrath. If the serous humour is corrupt, they are subject to evil passions and dreadful nightmares. Those with a predominance of bilious humour are generally slothful, given to bodily pleasures, sleepy, idle, dull of wit, heavy and slow. They love delicate food and drink. Those dominated by the atrabilious humour are hard to please, obstinate, suspicious, sorrowful and given to fearful thoughts.

The humours are exceedingly variable in quantity and quality. The sanguineous reigns from 3 am to 9 am; bilious from 9 am to 3 pm; serous from 3 pm to 9 pm and atrabilious from 9 pm to 3 am. The sanguineous humour increases in the spring. The heat of summer dissolves superfluities, wastes the humours and opens the pores. The breath escapes from the body with exhalations, moisture and vapors. The bilious humour is in ascendancy. Autumn breeds the serous humour.

Winter thickens the humours, constrains the sinews and sends natural heat inward. The atrabilious humour increases and makes people sluggish.

The active elemental qualities—cold and heat—form the humours. When heat is equable, the sanguineous humour forms; when heat is in excess, bilious humour forms; when in great excess so that oxidation occurs, atrabilious humour forms. When the cold is equable, serous humour forms; when cold is in excess so that congelation becomes dominant, atrabilious humour forms.

In addition to this, there are three souls within the human form:

> . . . namely, the vegetable, animal and rational, all of which descend from the world above and each of which possesses its own faculties. The more refined the mixture of the humours the greater the perfection and the more complete and perfect the possibility of receiving the soul. Moreover, in each man, health means the harmony of the humours and illness the disruption of the balance of the constitution. Of course the harmony is never perfect in any person, but relative to his own constitution, health means the re-establishment of the balance of the humours. Diagnosis for such disorders as fever are, in fact, based on searching for the way in which the balance of the humours has been upset. But for diseases which show overt signs, the most notable sign or signs are made use of it for diagnostic purposes and often the disease receives the name of the leading sign connected with it.[11]

Flowing in the space intermediate between the physical body and the force of life, is a placeless space, a space that, as a whole, has a direction and must have a center, the position toward which it is directed. Health or lack of it is is out from this center.

The Breath

The breath acts as the link between the body, soul and spirit. It is the breath which makes the perfect equilibrium of the elements possible.

God created the left side of the heart and made it hollow in order that it should serve both as a storehouse of the breath and as the seat of manufacture of the breath. He also created the breath to enable the drives of the "soul' to be conveyed into the corresponding members. In the first place the breath was to be the rallying-point for the faculties of the soul and in the second place it was to be an emanation into the various members and tissues of the body (whereby these could manifest the functions of those drives).

Now He produced the breath out of the finer particles of the humours and out of igneity and at the same time produced the tissues themselves (the visible body) out of the coarser and earthy particles of these humours. In other words, the breath is related to the attenuated particles as the body is related to the coarser particles of the same humours. Just as the humours are intermingled to produce a temperamental "form," whereby the members of the body are enabled to receive a physical appearance, impossible were they separate, so the attenuated portions of the humours, being intermingled into a temperamental form, enable the breath to receive the powers of the soul—impossible were the humours separate.

The beginning of the breath is as a divine emanation from potentiality to actuality proceeding without intermission or stint until the form (preparation, state) is completed and perfected. Each member, though derived from the self-same substance of the humours, nevertheless has its own particular temperament—for the proportional qualities of the (denser portions of the) humours and the form of their commixture are peculiar to each member. Similarly, although derived from the same attenuated portions of the humours, nevertheless each of the three breaths (natural, animal and vital) has its own particular temperament, because the proportional quantities of the more attenuated portions of the humours and the manner of their commixture are peculiar to each breath.

Although the body consists of several organs, there is one from which they all originally arose. As to what this organ actually was, there are various opinions. The fact remains that one organ necessarily came to light before other organs could arise out of it. Exactly the same is true in the case of the breaths. There is one single breath which accounts for the origin of the others. This breath, according to the most important philosophers, arises in the heart, passes thence into the principal centers of the body, lingering in them long enough to enable them to impart to it their respective temperamental properties. Lingering in the cerebrum it receives a temperament whereby it is capable of receiving the drives of sensation and movement; in the liver, it receives the drive of nutrition and growth (vegetative drives); in the generative glands it acquires a temperament which prepares it for receiving the drive of generation (reproduction).

The breath is similar to the spirit and is of three kinds:

(1) The vital spirit, hot and dry, has its center in the left ventricle of the heart, preserves life, causes the body to grow, move and reproduce, and travels through the arteries. (2) The psychic spirit, cold and wet, has its center in the brain, causes sensation and movement and moves through the nerves and is the source of movement and reason. (3) The natural spirit, hot and wet, has its center in the liver, is concerned with the reception of food, growth and reproduction and travels through the veins.[12]

Traditional medicine is first concerned with the rhythmic continuity of the breath itself and then the synthesis of breath as "time in motion" or "active space" and organs or members as "passive possibilities of space" of matter and form. Harmonic order brings together those two concepts of breath and organs which appear to be opposite but which inwardly contain one another and are therefore complements. The synthesis is achieved because the breath occupies a continuous space defined by passageways, meridians, channels which move through the shapes of organs, bones, muscles. Movement coalesces breath and organs into a unity.

The Organs

The humours in turn act as the constituent elements for the members or organs of the body which "are derived primarily from the commingling of the humours, just as the humours are derived primarily from the commingling of the aliments and the aliments are primarily composed of commingled elements. The organs are divided into simple ones having homogeneous parts such as flesh, bones, and nerves, and compound organs such as the hands and face. The organs are the instruments by which the passions and actions of the mind are achieved and act as its servants.

The primary elemental quality of an organ is based on its nutrient while its secondary quality is determined by what it excretes.

Hot organs consist of the vital force and heart, blood, liver, flesh, muscle, spleen, kidneys, breasts, testicles, muscular coats of arteries, veins, skin of palm (which is evenly balanced).

Cold organs consist of phlegm, hair, bones, cartilage, ligaments, serous membranes, nerves, spinal cord, brain, solid and liquid fats and skin.

Moist organs consist of phlegm, blood, sold and liquid fats, brain, spinal cord, breast, testicles, lungs, liver, spleen, kidneys, muscles, and skin.

Dry organs consist of hair, bones, cartilage, ligaments, tendons, membranes, arteries, veins, motor nerves, heart, sensory nerves, skin.

The Efficient Causes

> The efficient (*failiya*) causes are capable of either preventing or inducing change in the human body. They may be external to the person or internal. External causes are: age, sex, occupation, residence, and climate and other agents which effect the human body by contact whether contrary to nature or not. Internal causes are sleep and wakefulness, evacuation of secretions and excretions, the changes at different periods of life in occupation, habits and customs, ethnic group and nationality.

The efficient causes are clear and vary with each individual. Whereas the elements, humours, breath and organs as the material cause are all from nature, the efficient causes develop out of the nurturing process.

The Formal Causes

> The formal (*suriyah*) causes are three: temperaments (*mizajat*) (or the pattern of constitution as a whole) and the faculties or drives (*qawa*) which emerge from it and the structure (the quantitative patterns).

Temperament

Temperament arises from the elements and humours and it determines the way in which the soul functions. Each animal and each organ of the body has a temperament of its own.

> The Almighty Creator has bestowed upon every animal and every one of its organs the most appropriate and the best adapted temperament for its various functions and passive states.
>
> Since the verification of this truth is a matter for philosophers and not physicians, we may accept that the human being has been bestowed a most befitting temperament and most appropriate faculty or drives for the various active and passive states in the body. Similarly, every organ and member is endowed with the proper temperament appropriate to its own functional requirement. Some He has made more hot, others more cold, others more dry and others more moist.

The temperament is “equable” when the contrary qualities are in perfect equilibrium, and out of harmony or “inequable” when the temperament tends toward a particular quality. Therapeutics, then, are based on the allopathic principle of contraries. That is, "cold" diseases can be cured by "hot" remedies and vice versa.

Avicenna then explains this method further:

> It is worth remembering that when a medicine is referred to as being evenly balanced, it does not mean that its temperament is the same as of a human being, or that it is even similar to it, for it would then be like a human being. It merely means that such a medicine, after being acted upon by the innate heat [metabolized] fails to produce any material change in the normal state of the body, and that its pharmacological actions remain within the limits of normal human temperament. In other words, when this medicine is given to a normal person, it does not produce any appreciable change or imbalance in the body. When it is said that a drug is hot or cold, it does not mean that the physical quality of the drug is particularly hot or cold or that it is colder or hotter than the human body. If this were so there would follow the unwarranted inference mentioned above that an evenly constituted medicine is the one which has exactly the same temperament as the human body. It means just that such a medicine produces a greater amount of heat or cold than what was originally present in the body. A drug which, for example, is cold for the human being may be hot for the scorpion, or the medicine which is hot for the human being may be cold for the serpent. In fact it may also mean that the same medicine may be less hot for one person than for another. This is the reason why physicians are advised to change their medicine when it fails to produce the desired result.

The growth and decay of the human body is dependent upon the human temperament. Growth depends upon the heat contained in the sperm which is gradually used up. Meanwhile, the moisture lessens in quantity and quality, thus preserving the innate heat at a constant level up to the old age. Ultimately, however, the moisture of the body comes to an end, and the innate heat i.e. extinguished, thus causing the death to which everyone is destined and which depends upon the original temperament of the human body.

The correspondences between the various orders of reality and the temperament have been summed up in the following:

> The uniqueness of the temperament of each individual indicates that each microcosm is a world of its own, not identical with any other microcosm. Yet, the repetition of the same basic humours in each constitution bears out the fact that each microcosm presents a morphological resemblance to other microcosms. Moreover, there is an analogy between the human body and the cosmic order, as shown by the correspondence between the humours and elements. There is in the Hermetico-alchemical natural philosophy, which was always closely tied

to medicine in Islam, a basic doctrine of the correspondence between all the various orders of reality: the intelligible hierarchy, the heavenly bodies, the order of numbers, the parts of the body, the letters of the alphabet which are the "elements" of the Sacred Book, etc. The seven cervical and the twelve dorsal vertebrae correspond to the seven planets and the twelve signs of the Zodiac, as well as to the days of the week and the months of the year; and the total number of discs of the vertebrae, which they consider to be twenty-eight, to the letters of the Arabic alphabet and the stations of the moon. There is, therefore, both numerical and astrological symbolism connected with medicine, although the closeness of the relation has not been the same during all periods of Islamic history, nor among all the medical authorities. But the correspondence and "sympathy" (in the original sense of the word "sympathia") between various orders of cosmic reality form the philosophical background of Islamic medicine.[13]

The Faculties or Drives

The body also possesses faculties which originate the functions of various organs. The major faculties are (1) the vital (*hayawaniyah*), responsible for preserving the integrity of the breath, sensation, and movement of the heart; (2) the natural (*tabiiyah*) governing the nutritive powers of the liver and the reproductive powers of the generating organs; and (3) the animal (*nafsaniyah*) controlling the brain and the rational faculty.

The powers of the various members are due to the vital faculty[14] which provides the body with its inner force. The vital faculty is that which appears in the breath at the very moment at which the breath develops out of the rarefied particles of the humours.

Between the human body as a whole and the individual points as its parts there is a relationship—the whole being given with and active in the part and the part being aware that it is part and directly announcing its relation to the whole. Whenever we encounter a phenomenon showing this relationship between whole and parts we may assume, that a force, an ordered action of forces, is the basis. This is the role of the faculties which we can only know through their effects. They work through the physical body without ever touching it.

The Final Causes

The final (*tamamia*) causes are the actions or functions. They can be understood only from a knowledge of both the faculties or drives (*qawa*) and the vital energies (breaths, *arwah*) that are ultimately responsible for them. These will be described presently.

IV. Conclusion

The power of traditional Islamic medicine is in realizing that space leads and forms shapes; shapes then interact with space and space with the breath/inner light with which every human being has been endowed. What he or she does with that determines the extent of their completion and perfection.

O. Cameron Gruner's Remarks

During the past fifty years,[1] the popular imagination has been stirred by a succession of important discoveries in the domain of medicine and surgery. The triumphs of the latter field have been spectacular to a degree. Those of medicine have been much less conspicuous, chiefly because the mind must inquire into them before it can properly appreciate them. How much does not humanity owe to the steadily continued researches in bacteriology, and the painstaking observations which have revealed the life-cycles of many of the parasites to which tropical and other diseases are due and to the whole procedure of immuno-therapy, the just pride of scientific as distinct from clinical medicine, and the outcome of all these researches?

As compared with all this, the speculative subtleties of former times appear both futile and unworthy of resuscitation. But the ancient system was not as valueless as is so generally supposed. Taking as an adequate criterion the first book of *The Canon of Medicine* of Avicenna, which is here presented [almost in its entirety], and is fairly representative of the whole work, we find in its pages references to many departments of human knowledge—(though it might be objected that all these departments of knowledge are now separate sciences, each requiring its own professorial staff, its own literature, and journals and that they are not mentioned under the special names with which we are familiar, their existence in those days cannot be denied) cosmology, anatomy, physiology, and psychology; the: various branches of clinical medicine-etiology, semiology, diagnosis, and prognosis; the departments of therapeutics-hygiene, dietetics, balneology, and climatology, in addition to materia medica, pharmacology, and pharmacy. Moreover, the reader is presumed to be conversant with logic, criteriology, and metaphysics.

The presence of obvious literal errors in the work must not lead us to commit the more serious mistake of overlooking the fact that it is entirely built up upon a sound philosophy of human nature, which is as vitally important today, though largely ignored in former times. The traditional medicine was concerned essentially with the given patient now before us; whereas now it is simply the science of diseases which it is our duty to diagnose accurately, prevent if possible, and treat on lines capable of wholesale application. To Avicenna, the determination of the constitution of the patient was of the very first importance, because on it depended the character, course, and duration of his illness, and upon that again depended the choice of remedies.

After all, from the patient's point of view, the real object of consulting a medical man is to be restored to a state of well-being. It is little comfort to be virtually told that 85-90 percent of cases of his complaint are cured by the treatment adopted in his case, only to find that he proves to be one of the remaining 10-15 percent for whom there is little or nothing to be done. True, his sighs are drowned in the shouts of the fortunate, and fail to reach the clinical laboratory, surgical wards, consulting room or research councils.

If, in the interests of these few, chance leads us to the pages of this traditional work, it would seem that suggestions occur in it which enable us to understand their plight, and thereby help them to understand it also. Even if the enemy is not put out of action, his enmity is less evident when he is understood.

It has been the aim of this treatise to elaborate Avicenna's central theme by references to the various philosophies extant in his time—Sufi, Vedantic, Buddhist, Chinese; to Persian writings subsequent to his time (Rumi, Sadi, Shabistari, etc.); and to views presented by various modern philosophies, including western theosophy.

But these various directions of thoughts are not drawn upon in order to elaborate a composite system after the fashion of theosophical eclecticism. On the contrary, readers accustomed to various modes of thought are invited across a bridge leading from their various starting-points, across the chasm of modernism, until they reach the concise teaching of Thomistic philosophy, wherein all other aspects of the one truth receive their proportionate places. The inclusion of ideas from writers whose ideas appear to be altogether of the by-ways may torment a few, but may also help a few to see the: greater thing, and thereafter be content to stay upon the broad highway to which the several paths have converged.

Science has been removed from its usual role of master, and has been pressed into service, and that service is to illuminate the subject of human nature. To quote a recent paper,[2] "Under the great swelling flood that represents the growing complexity of modern medicine, let us not allow ourselves hold fast to that great life-saving conception of the essential unity of the human body. Let us oppose fearlessly those currents of medical thought that tend to isolate—arbitrarily and to the detriment of true knowledge—the various segments of this one great subject. Let us welcome all methods, all discoveries, that help the one man in charge of the one patient to broaden the base of his attack, to widen the sweep of his beneficent vision." These words were possibly expressed with a different object, but apply well to the theme of this treatise.

The old teaching about "constitution" should undergo a mutual intergrowth with the knowledge of modern science, pervaded throughout with the fundamental teaching of Thomistic philosophy, when there would emerge the beginnings of a possible system of modern scholastic medicine—thoroughly logical, plain, free of mystery, free of materialism, but not ignoring the so-called "occult" and metaphysical; with the knowledge of the nature of the constitution of the individual patient as its central and dominant theme. Were the whole medical training along such lines, the student would be able to approach his clinical instruction thoroughly aware that the individuality of the patient comes first, and that the ailment from which he suffers is but part and parcel of one single story, and not merely an accidental superposition. But the student would constantly need guidance to ensure his over-riding the disregard or ignorance, if not actual rejection, of scholastic principles which characterizes the concrete modern teaching of pathology in its various departments.

The following brief survey of the most important teachings of *The Canon*.

Teachings of The Canon

The General Notion of the Nature of a Human Being

The following three propositions belong to it: (1) the human being (MF)[3] is composed of matter and a principle of life, the two together making him "he" or "she," he or she is "a single substance endowed with a natural tendency to realize and maintain the conditions of its organization." (2) This principle of life comprises three main groups of potential and actual activities—the vegetative, the sensitive and the rational. This multi-potentiality of the principle of life is represented in the expression "bundle of life." (3) The organs of the body are the material manifestations (the actualities) of the several potentialities The vegetative organs belong to the "vegetative soul," the sense-organs and appurtenances belong to the "sensitive soul." The intelligence and will belong to the "rational soul," which has not literal organs but acts through the instrumentation of the organs of the vegetative and sensitive systems. All these components belong intimately together apart from macroscopic or microscopic boundaries it.

These propositions are further defined by the following negative statements: (1) the human being is not a collection of molecules and forces; he manifests chemical, electric, and other phenomena, which are not causes, but effects. (2) The organs are not distinct from the powers they exhibit. (3) The brain is not the producer of thought.

The remarkable action which the human being achieves by his complicated mechanical contrivances are distinct from himself, whereas in the human being the mechanism and the manipulator are the self same. Even when there is as grave mechanical interference with organs as occurs in hemiplegia, or in the cortical lesions of insanity, the rational soul remains untouched, though no longer able to communicate its activities to the outer world. To quote from St. Thomas, "The intellect, being a power that does not make use of a corporeal organ, would in no way be hindered in its act through the lesion of a corporeal organ, if for its act there were not required the act of some power that does make used of a corporeal organ."[4]

Thought is produced by the activity of the rational souls; the changes in the brain—whether chemical, cytological, or otherwise—are not causes, but the visible effects of the activity. (4) There is no bridge over the gulf between rational life and the-vegetative sensitive life; the distinctions are radical. (5) The life-principle is not subject to the laws of inheritance, those which govern matter; it is not divisible into organs, or parts, or elements. As soon as it ceases to operate, it is left behind the material body, which though apparently the same is actually quite different from the animate person recently before me.

The Notion of the Constitution of Any Given Individual When in Health

This notion should be made as tangible as possible.[5] The constitution may be expressed in terms of a number of formula to be taken together—a series of "notes," some of which are constants, and others variables. In this formula, the qualities are represented by the initials of their corresponding names; the quantities are represented by index numbers from 1 to 5, to stand for slight, moderate, normal, marked, and very marked, and very marked respectively.

The Constants

I. *The Body:* (1) general physique [good, poor, robust, spare, strong, delicate]; (2) dominant "element" [example: $E^2W^2F^5A^3$] for earth, water, fire and air; (3) dominant "humour," shown in the humoural formula [example: $S^3L^1B^5A^8$] for sanguineous, serous (lymphatic), bilious, and atrabilious]. This formula is really descriptive of the "temperament," but the latter word bears a different meaning in modern popular usage. (4) The absolute or relative strength or weakness (functional capacity) of the several organs; hypo, hyper-function. [example: $V^4T^4M^2O^3N^1G^3$, for vegetative (i.e. alimentary), thoracic (i.e. respiratory and circulatory), muscular (including skeletal), osseous (including genito-urinary), nervous (including sympathetic system) and glandular (including haemopoietic, endocrine, and hepatic) types. (5) The emotional make-up, or formula [example: $G^3L^2T^1I^5$ (gaudium, laetitia, timor, ira),[6] from which the dominant passion and its modifiers are noted. The modern use of the word "temperament" belongs here.

The difference in capacity is partly explained by considering the time-factor,[7] and partly as a fundamental difference.[8] All the material brought to an organ, whether nutritive, or excretory, is not at once taken up in its entirety; only a certain proportion is removed and the remainder passes on, so that the blood has its composition at a certain level. The modern threshold values recognize this fact. The time-factor is of very great importance.

II. *The Mind:* here comes the description of the disposition, the type of mind, or mental make-up.[9] Mental capacity may be expressed in terms of the relative or absolute strength or weakness of the various faculties, enumerated under "talents" (which are simply developments of particular faculties above the average).[10]

> "The better the disposition of a body, the better the soul allotted to it which clearly appears in things of different species: and the reason thereof is that act and form are received into matter according to matter's capacity thus because some men have bodies of better disposition, their souls have a greater power of understanding . . . . This occurs in regard to the lower powers of which the intellect has need in its operation, because those in whom the imaginative, cogitative and memorative powers are of better disposition, are better disposed to understand."[11]

The mental attitude towards things, which emerges from the character, is also to be noted, for sometimes this may explain the cause of the illness (i.e., wanton exposure to infections in spite of warnings), and will show whether the patient is suppressing relevant facts, will respond to treatment, or is secretly concerned with some fear or doubt which is the real object of his visit to the doctor. Moreover, knowledge of this aspect of character will safeguard the physician himself, either by making him aware of the patient's possible cynical opinion about a profession he is unfortunately obliged to deal with, or, more important, by enabling him to avoid offering advice which is palpably foolish to an intelligent patient.

The Variables

The degree of vitality: this is also spoken of as the strength of innate heat in the text;[12] (2) deviations from the functional capacities normal to the individual; (3) the nature or degree of "resistance." In terms of *The Canon*, this would be expressed in the "humoural formula," and in terms of "obstructions" of various kinds. These account for the "soil" which renders declared disease: (a) possible; or (b) amenable to alteration by artificial means.[13]

Foreign though such data are to modern clinical work, they are often actually employed in ordinary conversation, as when one describes a person as sanguine, or bilious, or phlegmatic, or as of saturnine temperament. Some adjective descriptive of the emotional make-up is not infrequent in case reports degrees of vitality are spoken of seriously by the laity, diplomatically by the practitioner.

In so far as they provide a simple means of codifying tentative knowledge upon complex and elusive individual characteristics which it is our duty to notice, the data are all worth consideration.

The Notion of the Nature of the State of Disease

The vegetative processes associated with digestion and absorption of food may be first briefly referred to. The picture of the whole nutritive cycle is comprehended in the idea of the "liver."[14] We trace the food constituents through the columnar cells of the intestinal mucosa, across the areolar tissue into the vascular roots of the portal and lacteal system; then into the liver unit itself (comprising phagocytic secretary cells, fundal cells, cubical excretory cells, and the hepatic arterioles and lymphatic clefts related to the sinusoids); then into the general blood-stream, and finally out of the body through various organs, including the goblet cells of the intestinal mucosa, the bile-ducts, the pancreas, etc. The extra-hepatic portion of the cycle is nearly co-terminous with the rest of the body.

To complete this picture we first remember the relation between the quality of food and the quality of chyme; then we consider how the ultimate components of the food travel (N-compounds, glucose, fat, phosphorus, sulphur, iron, and the like)—during rest, exercise, sleep, etc. and according to the character of the diet as a whole, the fluids taken, and the state of the bowels, etc. We may realize that they are manifested in the blood in the form of alkaline tide, viscosity, fibrin-content, and the various morphological changes revealed by blood-examination. We picture also the innumerable chemical interchanges and physical transformations in various parts of the cycle; the formation of waste-substances, and the factors on which the whole of the processes depend. [15] In brief, then our picture of the body is that of a complex of tubes and channels —potential as well as actual—which vary in size from the obvious alimentary-canal, air-passages, and great blood vessels, down to the finest ramifications of the latter, the cavernous tissues—both macroscopic and microscopic—the serous cavities, and the intracellular channels. All these form one continuous labyrinthine system, through which we may trace the ingested food materials, the metabolic, secretory and excretory products. As long as these channels are patent throughout, and As long as these various subs stances (including the "breath of life") can flow freely through them, and the vital energy has a free play outward, so long is the body in a state of health.

But as soon as there is a continued interference with the freedom of movement, even though it be merely an ebb and flow that is affected, in any part of the canalicular system, then a state of disease arises, culminating in histological anatomical changes. Hence, when we observe a case of illness, we may be sure there is some "obstruction" in some channels in some part of the body—not necessarily in that where the symptoms occur (i.e., the nasal discharge of "cold in the head," the bronchial expectoration in bronchitis, the serous effusion into the pleura, the respiratory phenomena in an attack of asthma, are manifestations in the respiratory system of obstructions elsewhere).

The next addition to the picture of the sick person's state is furnished by the causes of the obstruction. Avicenna considered these under two groups, the '"material" (i.e. those in which "matter" is concerned) or "humoural diseases" and the non-material. To the latter group would belong cases of gross obstruction, such as by compression from without, or such as by obstruction with calculi and those in which there is a functional disorder—hypo-function, hyper-function, dysfunction. For instance, in renal disease, the loss of functional capacity may render the-normal ebb and flow of substances disorderly.[16]

The group of humoural diseases is predominant in Avicenna's pathology, and if we bear in mind what the "humours" really are, this position becomes quite reasonable. Perverted metabolism is associated with changes of physical state in the fluids of the body. Limpid fluids may become viscid, viscous substances may become mobile or "tenuous." In the ancient work, these chemical changes were thought of, not in "equations," but under interchanges between the imponderable elements, as being subject to the laws of *uruj, nasul, jalal, jamal, qada, qadr*,[17] the rhythm, phases and rate of movement of the "breath" and the fluctuations of degrees of innate heat. Concrete examples are such as: precipitation of urates in tissues, altered reaction of tissue juices in rheumatoid arthritis, cardio-renal disease, tuberculosis; variations of content of Ca, Na, Mg, etc., in the tissue-water, so that the flow from tissue to blood and vice versa is impeded.[18]

The Canon often insists on the presence of "superfluities" as a cause of "obstructions" of the canalicular system not only in the tangible four humours, but also in regard to the "breath."[19] In the latter case, the substance of the breath (i.e. water-vapor) ceases to be "bright," and "clear," and its odor becomes offensive, and its freedom of flow is impaired .

Finally, adding from modern knowledge, there are the changes in the fluids of the body produced by bacterial or putrefactive breakdown—whether this begins in intestinal stasis or arises in the course of specific bacterial infections. There are then obstructions not only in the old sense, but in the form of the successive histological lesions consequent—vascular, nutritional, and inflammatory. Materials are deposited more or less permanently (irreversible reactions), as i.e., solid odema, collagenous tissue, scar formation, fibrosis, and hyalo-fibrosis, adipose tissue, hyperplastic formations. Loss of anatomical patency is super added to loss of functional perviousness.

Clearly, whereas we give first place to the bacterial invasion, Avicenna gave it to the habits of life. He was deeply impressed by the obvious fact that the quality of food determines the kind of chyme, and that the kind of chyme determines the quality of the freedom of flow through the diffuse canalicular system of the body. As they accumulate in the stagnating tissue-juices they come to exercise a noxious action; they come to be beyond the capacity of the third and fourth digestions (tissue-digestion), and with their stagnation, the ever-circulating bacteria (taken up with the food) also settle and multiply and wandering-cell infiltrations gather together. The beginnings of disease are laid down. The functional disturbance has been succeeded by anatomical lesions.[20]

Finally, Avicenna enlarges his view of humoural disease by noting the influence of many extracorporeal factors[21] as well as the period of life, not to mention "the decree of God."[22] Thus, one and the same kind of food taken at the "warm" period of life in the "warm" season may contribute more to the formation of a given humour than at another.

If we knew the patient's formula, and how the climactic and other conditions are likely to affect it, and whether they are compatible or not with susceptibility to the agents at work, our composite picture of the patient's state would be of great value, and illnesses often inexplicable would lose their mystery. How much more efficient might not the treatment be, if the remedial measures in contemplation were selected to harmonize with them?

No doubt only a fanatic would note the barometer, thermometer, humidity, hours of sunshine, wind-direction and velocity, the character of previous seasons, the clues afforded by then migration so insects, rodents, and birds, the presence or prevalence of certain parasites in a district, and the many other points noted in Part Three[23] before prescribing the regimen for the patient. But it would seem that some Eastern physicians of bygone times conscientiously strove to learn from such factors.

The Guides to the Diagnosis of the State of the Patient

The patient before us is as a manuscript written in some highly complex language which it is our business to decipher. The alphabet is furnished by the several colors, the simple observations of size, shape, consistency, contour, texture, and the like. The vocabulary consists of the external features both in repose and animation, and of the physical signs as taught to-day. The grammar lies in the "general guides" (sphygmology, urinoscopy, examination of feces and blood). The language is to be translated into: states of natural (vegetative), sensitive, and emotional instinctive drives, functional capacities, plethora, obstructions, solutions of continuity, etc. that is, the state of the whole composite, in all aspects. This task can only be accomplished imperfectly at the best, even by the most skilled and most learned. Our silent teachers, or guides, the "indications" always enable us to ascertain something, and we must perforce be content with that on the present occasion and be determined to use this experience as the guide to better success on the next.

One of the guides suggested in *The Canon* lies in one's own state of health. Properly to interpret what we observe, we must ourselves have no disharmony of functions arising from errors of diet, no deposit in the urine, no weight in the bowels, no obstructions in our own brain, no mental fatigue, no emotional pre-occupation, no rigid notions regarding etiology or prognosis; there must be clear channels for the breath, and the breath must be under the control of the will. It must be kept pure by recollection, by devotion, and observance of prayer. The reason for this is that under such conditions, long persevered, we are enabled to receive an "impression" from the patient. We become aware of his atmosphere, aura, or personality in the form of an idea of his degree and kind of vitality. But unless this impression is registered rapidly, namely at the first approach of the patient, it will be confused and illegible by reason of the mutual inter-impression of one's own vitality with his. In another idiom, we observe "with the eye of a Taoist." In our own idiom, we make use of sound reasoning power, common sense, and a certain kind of "intuition," or "clinical sense."

The guides furnished by general observation of the patient are, in brief: (1) external features in repose: (a) colors of face, hair, skin, eye (sclerae, iris); (b) odors and savors; (c) form of the body: (i) as a whole; (ii) in detail. The features, the hands, the limbs; the relative proportions (length, breadth, and thickness) of nose, cheeks, upper lip, lower lip, chin, mouth, ears, orbit, eyebrows, forehead, etc.; the character of the neck, shoulders, etc. (2) Features when animated: (a) expression, gaze, look, facial gestures (vivacity, sleepiness, languidness); (b) deportment or attitude,24 gestures, carriage, specific acts or mannerisms, definitely morbid movements or defective movements. (c) voice: tone of voice, manner of speech (clear, loud, or the opposite); clues to the physical and mental type, and the degree of energy and vitality.

Space does not allow of any attempt to furnish precise details of the external signs of functional capacity of internal organs. The principle is exemplified thus: the lower part of the nose is part of the respiratory system, and shares in the degree of development of the whole system; therefore wide nostrils with well-formed aloe go with good development of the whole respiratory function, whereas narrow delicate nostrils and small alae refer the observer to some other system as well-developed. Large mouth, thick lips, large masseters, and generally well-developed lower part of the face go with good development of the digestive tract throughout. Moreover, development or capacity above the average in one system denotes relative weakness and functional deficiency in another system. The subject is extensive.[25]

Our general guides differs noticeably, from that revealed in *The Canon*. To follow Avicenna, (1) when one places the hand on the pulse, one absorbs oneself in it, without the distraction of a watch, until one has found out how it runs minute after minute. Even if it misses, without an intermission of the heart, because the patient gives a twitch of the finger or begins to talk, one learns even from that. The study of the circulation is more than the study of the heart's action. (2) When one examines the urine, even with all the apparatus of modern chemistry, we must remember that it is first and foremost the guide to the state of digestion—especially its "second stage" (that in the liver) as well as in the "third" stage (that in the small vessels). We are misled by the search for albuminuria and glycosuria, for many would make these abnormalities into diseases. Thus, the number of persons in whom albuminuria is not evidence of renal disease far outnumber those in which it is; the presence of such a substance in the urine should lead to the questions: is some substance not being dealt with? If so, why? Can only the kidney handle it? To follow a useful rule, the real trouble is remote. It may lie in the brain, in the emotional state (cf. Graves' disease, i.e., pentosuria, cystinuria, alkaptonuria also break the current ideas about urinalysis.[26] (3) As regards the guide furnished by the feces matter, again, our knowledge is much greater than was Avicenna's and we do not apply it in his terms. We are apt to lose ourselves in fat analyses, nitrogen estimations, occult blood tests, B. coli classifications. Negative results in each case are taken to mean nothing of note, regardless of the continual secretory and excretory changes proceeding in the intestinal mucosa, and the vitality of nerve-ganglia, etc. Essential and definite derangements may occur without conspicuous deviations from the restricted standards usually laid down.

The guide furnished by an examination of the brood may be spoken of as the most notable modern addition to Avicenna's three general guides. The data obtained from it—physical, physicochemical, cytological, serological—are very numerous, but are lost more often than not by restriction to the diagnosis of the various "blood-diseases." When properly applied, all the data obtained from the blood inform us of the functional state of all the organs and of the existence of the main groups of pathological state.[27]

The Relation Between *The Canon* and Modern Thought

Considerations[37] are not wanting which entitle The Canon of Medicine of Avicenna to an esteemed position in modern thought. In the first place, there is the outstanding intellectual culture of the [Islamic] Empire—during the period of history to which Avicenna belongs. Secondly, in the case of much of his teaching, it may be said that the difference from ours is largely only that his speech is alien and is apt to be misunderstood. In these days, the great complexity of the language with which we express our scientific thought corresponds with the intricacy of the instruments wherewith facts are elicited. Thirdly, many of the advances of modern times offer the solutions to the very theorems and propositions of former times. Finally, ideas are to be found in his work which provide suggestions for useful research in the future.

The importance of idea over material achievement is not to be forgotten. The achievements of any age are subject to decay with the lapse of centuries but the ideas which gave rise to them remain living through all cycles. Therefore to propose a real place for Avicenna in modern thought is not to propose a return as it were to old architecture, or the costumes of long ago. It is rather to render accessible today the picture which he painted and so enable it to renew its still vital message. It is to play over again the music which he expressed and enable perhaps one or two to rejoice in it. And this without obscuring the issue by discussing nationality or schools of thought or evolution of ideas or technical methods.

If it appear to some a fault that the master appears to have used passages from other works and this without full acknowledgment, it should be remembered that after all a painter may use pigments which someone else has manufactured and is allowed even to employ other persons (usually pupils) to execute certain portions of his picture. Indeed, even after his decease, it is not improper that some may have been entrusted with the delicate task of touching up faded portions of the canvas which he bequeathed.

The place for Avicenna in modern thought is gained when it is agreed that he shall be viewed as one who entered this world entrusted with a mission independently to express for that age, by means of those various tools which he then found in it, the wisdom which is unchanging and impersonal. So also there is the need today that this same wisdom should be re-expressed for this age by means of the new data which lie to our hands.

The Nature of the Knowledge Presented by *The Canon*

The Canon is a precis and not a sum-total of Avicenna's knowledge. Numerous passages occur in *The Canon* which show that this is the case, that it is a series of notes or skeleton outlines of thought not too lengthy to be memorized by his students[52] much as they would memorize the Quran. Thus, "to the full extent necessary, and yet with apt brevity,"[53] "do not place in medicine what does not belong to it,"[54] "having discussed the equable temperaments sufficiently,"[55] "I purposely omit reference to certain other problems relative to the fluids of the body just as much as is necessary to enable you to practice medicine intelligently."[56] Many passages also refer to others of his own works for further details, to avoid confusing the purely medical issue of *The Canon*. These philosophical works are gradually becoming more widely known.

"Generally speaking, the saying of the saints and sages are terse, presenting only the germs of truth; these are developed by later teachers and then expanded and added to. We must see to it, however, that we get at the original meaning of the saints and sages."[57]

"Books are only words and the valuable part of words is the thought therein contained. That thought has a certain bias, which cannot be conveyed in words, yet the world values words as being the; essence of books. But though the world values them, they are not of value; as that sense in which the world values them is not the sense in which they are valuable."[58]

To say that a work is the product of the age in which an author lives is certainly often an error, for it is to confuse the person's insight with the tools (the language at his command) available to express himself with. Similarly to work out the relation between a literary work and the religious belief of the author, as for instance to show the relation between Islamic science and the Quran carries the same fallacy with it. The Prophet said, "Every soul when born is a faithful follower; it is afterwards that he becomes unfaithful"—which is to say that the form of religious belief is a secondary implantation, whereas the spirit of a sincere life can be traced to the original being.

Avicenna's medicine, like Indian medicine, has been traced to the Greek system. But it has been proved that the great works of *Charaka* and *Susruta* were available in Arabic, under the title of *Kitab shawshura al-Hindi*, from the 7th century.[59] Similarly, the view that the Chinese borrowed their philosophy of the five elements from the Turks has been sufficiently disposed of by Forke.[60] It is beside the purpose of this treatise to take up such questions.

The common notion that progress or stagnation in secular knowledge has a causal relationship with a certain religion is typically voiced in his address on "*Medicine and the Church*" by Sir Farquhar Buzzard.[61] The comment to make is: "*post hoc sed non propter hoc*." The advances in the science of medicine, as in all other sciences, are surely a part of the divine plan for mankind whereas the collateral abandonment of religious fundamentals remains a human responsibility.

The word "canon" (*qanun*): equivalent words: code of laws; series of principles; tao.[62] Principle is defined as "something antecedent, which exercises a real positive influence upon the consequent" = causes (four kinds, Avicenna) = reasons.

In view of this it is clear that *The Canon* is not properly to be regarded as an "encyclopedia" of the knowledge of the time, or to be contrasted, for instance, with the now classical "*Osler*."

The word "knowledge": knowledge is not simply an assemblage of "facts" nor is it to be made synonymous with "truth"—certainly not Absolute Truth, of which all human knowledge falls short although one single word is capable of containing or implying all knowledge, as in mathematics a single term may be equated with an infinite number of terms summed together. But even the mathematical sciences can only afford approximate truth.[63] We may recall the words, "If he attain to all knowledge, he is far off still."[64]

Facts, as St. Thomas[65] explains, are what our intellect regards as external objects—and as we judge of them only in terms of our sense organs—these objects may be different. God knows them as they are. Our intellect depends on our imagination and that depends on our senses. Our senses only convey discrete fragments which we gather into one continuous impression regardless of intervening points." We live as it were in a network only the nodes of which are evident to the senses.

Mystical Insight

There is a distinction between knowledge gained in the ordinary manner and that gained by "mystical insight" (*kashf*). The writer of *Gulshan-i-raz's*[66] advises his readers to follow this, saying:

> Straightway lift yourself above time and space,
> Quit the world and be yourself a world for yourself.
> And
>
> The moment we are enlightened within
> We go beyond the voidness of a world confronting us.
> —Seng-ts'an, quoted by Susuki.[67]

As this "opens up all of a sudden a world hitherto undreamed of, it is an abrupt and discrete leaping from one plane of thought to another."[68]

> Real science is seeing the fire directly,
> Not mere talk, inferring the fire from the smoke.
> Your scientific proofs are more offensive to the wise
> Than the urine and breath whence a physician infers.[69]

"Man looks at the surface of the ocean. Yet he is so small that he cannot even be compared to one of its drops, limited as he is in intellect and in his knowledge. It is only to those who, having just touched creation, bow to God, forgetting their limited self, that God has remained. These through whom God has spoken are the only beings who have been able to give any truth to the world."[70]

"The mind is not like a horizontal door which haste be made larger by force. You must clear away the obstructions arising from creaturely desire and then it will be pure and clear with no limit to its knowledge. Heng Ch'u said, 'When the mind is enlarged it can enter into everything throughout the universe.' He who praises God knows about Him."[71]

This attitude towards nature is to be claimed for Avicenna on the plain evidence of his other writings including the *al-Najat* which appropriately appears in the Arabic version of *The Canon* printed at Rome in 1593 and of the Libellus on the powers of the hearts and is included in the Latin edition of *The Canon*, 1595.[72]

The acquisition of knowledge by this process demands nothing more than a keen observation of the life around us and was as much within his reach as ours. Such knowledge is not too restricted to one period of history, one language, or to one or two universities. And if it should seem that because our civilization is so different his opportunities were much less, we may pause to reflect that the difference between our age and his is chiefly one of mechanical appurtenances and phraseology; and that even to this day we need not travel far (i.e., the old streets of Cordova and Granada or more definitely, to northern Africa) to see much the same sort of scenery as he was accustomed to, much the same sort of life as is drawn in the 1001 Nights. In any case, what is human life, at bottom, but a matter of buying and selling, receiving and giving, seizing and relinquishing, constructing and demolishing, acquiring learning and losing it, seeking power and breaking it, bidding and forbidding, giving in marriage and seeking to obtain in marriage, birth and death.

The significant phrase "seeing into one's own nature,"[73] in which most admirable work occur many passages by way of explanation) gives a graphic description of that which gives Avicenna his superiority. *The Canon* is simply the medical garb in which the one Truth is expounded. It is for us also to perceive it in whatever idiom it might be described—western, eastern, Islamic, Confucian or Buddhist, for example.

It would then seem as if the mind were now able to float as it were round all the concepts the human being has ever given to the world, or round all the most familiar events of one's daily life, and perceive clearly that which can never be set forth in words. We should then also quote the words."[74] I perceive of it that it is something, but what it is I cannot perceive. Only it seems if I could conceive it, I should comprehend all truths.

Further than this, to find that some of the statements in *The Canon* are certainly erroneous and that modern investigations have placed us at an infinitely greater advantage, does not invalidate the work as a whole. Its possibilities for suggesting thoughts of real value today are more realized the more one reads between the lines, and the present treatise does not claim to exhaust them.

"Let not the authority of the writer offend thee, whether he be of title or great learning, but let the love or pure truth entice thee to read."[75]

Insight into eternal truths. A person may: (1) glimpse them; (2) understand them moderately; (3) understand them fairly thoroughly. But in describing them to another, he may explain them: (i) imperfectly (no one can explain them properly!); (ii) inadequately or incompletely; (iii) wrongly because of: (a) imperfect education; (b) educational bias; (c) religious or anti-religious bias; (d) inherently erroneous methods of thought; (e) restriction to logic. Such truths, again, may be denied by persons being told of them, for because in their turn they misunderstand, or understand only in part, either through careless attention, and (a) to (e).

Insight Versus Intuitional Knowledge

A note should here be made that the term "insight" as used here bears a rather different meaning to that pertaining to the term "intuitive knowledge," which St. Thomas[76] ascribes solely to the angelic mind, and defines as "the attainment of the truth of a thing at a single glance without the aid of reasoning."[77] On the other hand this mode of perceiving truths need not be disallowed a rudimentary commencement among the powers of the human soul, just as the "brute" mind must be allowed to contain rudiments of those high mental capacities which characterize the human being. Throughout all orders of creation, the lower are endowed with the scaffolding for the manifestation of successively more exalted capacities of the higher.

The Basic Difference between The Canon and Modern Medicine

The Canon treats of:

I. Speculative Medicine
   Certain fundamental principles (cosmology, psychology, metaphysics)

II. Practical Medicine

A. Application of Speculative Medicine to the study of (i) health; (ii) disease (tendency, predisposition, threshold stage, declared disease; (iii) cessation of life.
B. Actual treatment of "disease" by: (i) regimen, (ii) drugs, (iii) operative interference.

Modern Medicine consists of:
A. Principles of Medicine: The application of the facts of chemistry, physics, anatomy, biology to the systematic description of innumerable "diseases" classified as far as possible on the basis of the microbic theory; symptomatology; etiology; diagnosis.
B. Practice of Medicine
   i) Laboratory work
   ii) Therapeutics, Pharmacology and Dietetics
   iii) Surgery
   iv) Gynecology and Obstetrics
   v) States of Medicine: Hygiene in all its ranches
   vi) Psychological Medicine: Treatment of insanity
   vii) Legal medicine, etc.

Modern medicine is based on the conception of the universe as a conglomeration of dead matter out of which, by some unexplainable process, life may become evolved in forms. To Avicenna the whole of the universe is the manifestation of a universal principle of life, acting through the instrumentality of forms. Or, again, in modern medicine, the forms are the source of life; to Avicenna they are the product of life. Space itself is an aspect of the one life.[78]

In this way the difference between Avicenna's conception of "principles," and that of modern medicine is easily shown. To the school boy "science" would consist of (a) bookwork and (b) laboratory work which his teachers would insist is the basis of (a). Similarly, the medical curriculum begins with lectures, although these are more and more inclined to become laboratory demonstrations; and goes on to laboratory and hospital work.

In short, Avicenna's medicine, and all ancient and traditional medicine, is intimately bound up with philosophy, to wit, that of human nature—a philosophy which proves to be virtually identical with "modern scholastic philosophy," no doubt partly because the Quranic account of the origin of the human being tallies with the Christian.

Modern medicine, on the other hand, assuming the title and rank of a positive science, emphatically discards and excludes it. Hence we read: "the physiologist" (said Burdon Sanderson) "can pursue philosophy if he has a turn for it, but must understand that the moment he enters the field of philosophy he leaves his tools behind him." For "it is unfortunate that the limitations of scientific thought were often ignored by men of science in their writings . . . the result diverts those who know, but befogs the unsuspicious reader who will probably put the blame on his intelligence."[79]

"According to positivism, science cannot be as Aristotle conceived it, the knowledge of things through their ultimate causes, since material and formal causes are unknowable, final causes are illusions, and efficient causes are simply invariable antecedents, while metaphysics under any form is illegitimate."[80] Or, expressed more boldly, "philosophy" is considered to be the exact antithesis of the truth which modern medicine gives us, and is therefore inherently inadmissible to medicine.

The ignorance which accounts for this attitude is only met by insisting on proper definitions of terms. The following apply here:

Philosophy is "the science which is concerned with first causes and principles; it is the profound knowledge of the universal order, and the duties which that order imposes on the human being.[81]

Again, philosophy is the true perception and understanding of cause and effect. Metaphysics is "that portion of philosophy which treats of the most general and fundamental principles underlying all reality and all knowledge."[82] Psychology is "the science which treats of the soul and its operations" and, therefore, clearly, must be the real foundation of medicine.

It is in modern scholastic philosophy that the student finds ample exposure of the fallacy in positivism and its cognates, enabling him to detect the difference between false and true, expressed with enough force of logic to satisfy the most meticulous. This queen of all the sciences amply proves positivist science (including medicine) to be incomplete knowledge when taken alone. The knowledge of movement or change must be supplemented by mathematical and metaphysical viewpoints.[83] Such men as Albertus Magnus and Roger Bacon were convinced of the necessity of linking the sciences with philosophy.[84]

When medicine has in this way become ennobled it reaches its highest degree of perfection, in that it penetrates to the very depths of reality,85 admitting this knowledge to need, even then, a further complement to make it complete-namely, knowledge in relation to God ("Christian wisdom").

"Sapientia est scientia qua considerat causas primas et universales causas. Sapientia causas primas omnium causarum considerat."86 "Ille qui cognoscit causam altissimam simpliciter, qua est Deus dicitur sapiens simpliciter, in quantum per regulas divinas omnia potest judicare et ordinare."[87] *"Non acquiritur studio humano, sed est deursum scendens."*[88] *"Cum homo per res creatas Deum cognoscit, magis videtur hoc perti nere ad scientiam, ad quam perti net formaliter, qu am ad sapientiam ad qu am pertinet materialiter: et e converso cum secundum res divinas judicamus de rebus creatis, magis hoc ad sapientiam quam ad scientiam pertinet."*[89]

As St. Thomas said in his day, "they think that nothing exists besides visible creatures." [N.B.:"Creatures" are (a) animate; and (b) inanimate]. "They think that things proceed not by the divine will but by natural necessity."[90] So even in those days time and fortune were expended on researches which sound philosophy would have shown to be inherently futile.

We may reflect for instance on the reiterated search for a location of the soul, which the pioneer anatomists prosecuted, and also on the commonly repeated announcement to successive students of anatomy that the pineal gland is now no longer regarded as the site of the soul. There is the sub-conscious suggestion to the student that scientific research has effectively disposed of the medieval belief in the soul, whereas history only proves that the revolt against the precise teachings of the Council of Trent necessarily came to naught.[91] The very definition of "soul" which this council laid down makes a search for its location ludicrous.

Knowledge Common to Avicenna and Modern Medicine

A perusal of the text of The Canon will show many passages which apply quite well, without explanation, in these days. Thus, the following may be specified: the close relation between emotions and physiological states (shown to be even closer than modern research has realized); the classification of people into sanguine, phlegmatic, bilious, saturnine, frigid, "hot"; the physiology of sleep; and how posture may remedy insomnia.

Choice of Location for Dwellings

Health resorts. Climactic influences on health and illness- Plethoric maladies. Dietetics. Hydrotherapy. Regiminal treatment. The uses of counter-irritation. Bier treatment. The introduction of remedies into the urethra. The use of vaginal tampons. The use of anesthetics by the mouth (medicated wines: scopolamine). Testing the strength of a drug by animal experiment. The treatment of insanity by malaria.[124]

No doubt the great difference between the ancient and modern is one of outlook, which accounts for the difference of topic. That which appeared interesting and even important in those days is passed over by modern physiology and pathology. Each century has its own interests. The mistake made is to suppose that the older interests were "wrong," "incorrect," "useless"; and to label them as "out of date." True, fashions of all kinds come to be out of date, but the epithets "right," "wrong" do not apply. The more carefully we observe modern science the more evident does it become that just its terminology and subject of conversation is different Things are seen from new angles, and things only surmised at then are amenable to tangible description now.

In fact, there occur moments, even at this day, when suggestive thoughts might be drawn from The Canon, to help in studying the individual, tedious, or baffling case, especially where the practice is far distant from the laboratories and appliances of modern medicine.

Of Interest to the Scholar

The present translation is based on the Latin versions published at Venice in 1608 and 1595, supported by a study of the Arabic edition printed at Rome in 1593 and the Bulaq edition.

It is true that as E. G. Browne pointed out, "The Latin Qanun swarms with barbarous words which are not merely transcriptions, but in many cases almost unrecognizable mistranscriptions of Arabic originals,"[125] and that Hirschberg and Lippert[126] regard the Latin as almost unintelligible, though they admit the "slavish adherence" of the Latin to the Arabic. Campbell[127] states that there was a "society of translators" at Toledo, about 1130 A.D., "whose method of translating from Arabic to Latin was to put the Latin equivalent over the Arabic words, disregarding the sense of the original." It is true that in many passages the obscurity is similar to the effect which would result if one were at this day to render idiomatic French word for word into English.

It is important to point out that the Latin of Volume I is very different from that of Vols. III-V; so different that the translation must have been the work of different persons. While the criticisms are justified with regard to these three volumes, they do not apply to the first, whose Latin is very close to the Arabic, and hardly to be improved. The difficulty really is that the Arabic itself is so condensed that the meaning can only be clearly represented in English by the use of many more words, whether to help out the meaning itself, or to make a presentable reading.

It may well be said, as did E. G. Browne, "He who judges Arabian Medicine only by the Latin translation will inevitably undervalue it and do it a great injustice. Indeed it is difficult to resist the conclusion that many passages in the Latin version of the *Qanun* of Avicenna were misunderstood or not understood at all by the translator, and consequently can never have conveyed a clear idea to the reader."[128]

The following aids to clearness have been utilized: (1) the study of Avicenna's other works, and of contemporary philosophical writings, in the existing translations. (b) The study of various Latin terms as understood by modern scholastic philosophy in its exposition of the medieval nomenclature. (c) The use of modern terms when there is no reasonable doubt of their referring to the same idea, though the literal term in the Latin is obsolete. The careful study of the original Arabic has here been of special importance, for words in the Latin version, which are evidently technical there, become merely colloquial when translated into English, whereas in the Arabic version, such words at once take on their proper character in the Arabic-English and Persian-English dictionaries (d) The use of tabulation of the matter. There are instances where this proves possible without omitting even a single Arabic word. (e) The use of paraphrase for certain passages. These are marked (p). A certain freedom of rendering has been inevitable in view of the importance of bringing the meaning of the text to the reader's notice without subjecting him to the need of reflecting deeply on passage after passage-as is requisite with the original Arabic (to have dealt with the work from the point of literature would have entailed giving the preference to safeguarding against likely criticisms at the hands of pure scholarship).

The main purpose of this treatise will now be seen to center in the idea that in the ancient philosophy there is material capable of useful application to-day. The selection of the work of Avicenna is not intended to provide an apologium for that one author, but is specially appropriate for these reasons: (i) his acknowledged excellence; (ii) his greater accessibility among medieval medical writings; (iii) a certain indefinable charm of expression peculiar to himself; but above all, (iv) the fact that his central theme is a conception of the nature of the human being really identical with that of Thomistic philosophy, and in these days specially stressed and developed by "modern scholastic philosophy." As these are related, so might Avicenna be related to a modern scholastic medicine, which would aim at reasons for health and ill health far deeper than those given by the microbic and cognate theories.

With Mercier,[129] "We do not regard the Thomistic philosophy . . . as a boundary which sets limits to personal activity of thought . . . but make use of his" (in this case, Avicenna's) "teaching as a starting-point from which we may go further afield."

With Maher,[130] we ". . . resuscitate and" (apply to medicine) ". . . a psychology that has already survived four and twenty centuries, and has had more influence on human thought and human language than all other psychologies together. My desire, however, has been not merely to expound, but to expand this old system . . . to make clear to the student of modern thought that this ancient and traditional psychology (and medicine) is not so absurd, nor these old thinkers as foolish, as current caricatures of their teaching would lead one to imagine. . . . To trespass (on the soul) . . . . is assumed by (many writers) to be the gravest of professional delinquencies."

Therefore Avicenna is allowed once more to present his theme. To the questions we are constrained to ask of him, we find our answers: (1) in his other writings; (2) in contemporary literature; (3) in the writings of modern Eastern thinkers; (4) in the works of St. Thomas; (5) in modern scholastic philosophy. If some truths are crudely expressed or perhaps faultily explained, it is our privilege to re-express and re-explain with those aids.

Those who may have failed to identify one single Truth under different garbs are not obliged to accord these garbs an unfriendly reception upon the stage of our modern world. To recall a favorite Indian metaphor, the danseuse has so robed herself, and displays such diversities of art that under the ever-changing colored beams of light it is difficult to believe there can be only one and the same artiste before us. Should it prove impossible to verify this, at least the very exhibition of the art should serve so to refresh that we can resume our work and ambitions with an added zest now confident that the future realization of our desires is not so intangible as at first appeared.

I deemed life was tranquillity and rest,
I find it but a never-ending quest;
And I, who sat in quietude and peace,
Toil on a journey that shall never cease
(Shamshad)

Why should the Cosmos turn its wheel of worlds
If not to search for Thee eternally?
Why should the tireless Sun arise each morn

If not to look for Thee?
(Zauq)

How can I win that Hidden One
Who sits within the secret place,
For even in my very dreams
She wears the veil upon Her face.
(Jurat)

For long, throughout the world, I sought for Thee,
Through weary years and ages of unrest—
At last I found Thee hidden in my arms
Within my breasts.
(Zauq)

That which is spread before us, beneath the unceasing surge and change of the crowded life of the thoroughfares of great cities, as well as beneath the panorama of nature herself, was surely understood by those who insisted " there is no second Cause," and by Chu Hsi in saying "the innumerable laws (of nature) all proceed from one source."[131] In this the thought is not pietistically of a Creator, but of a living Reality met (passively or receptively) or encountered (actively or contestingly) by us all at all times. That Reality must be understood before we handle the problem of our patient with real efficacy.

In the intention of this work, then, there comes into consideration that greater art of medicine—not an ethical Hippocratic ideal, but something of the divine—an art as real to Avicenna, philosopher, poet, musician, the worker among the great and the small, aware of the dramatic in life, as it should be to us. So we step out of the world of the modern critic, the scholar, and the medical historian, indeed of modern medicine itself, into one in which we stand, as it were, hand in hand, with the great Master of the East—almost with his very eyes gazing upon and scrutinizing this ever open book of life of ours—divested of the false notions of "progress" and "time." His language is thus no longer alien—and, incidentally, he lives again!

Avicenna's Preface

In the first place we render thanks to God, for the very excellence of the order of His creation, and the abundance of His benefits. His mercies are upon all the prophets. Secondly, is at the request of one of my special friends [was it al-Juzjani? LB], one whom I feel most bound to consider, that I prepare this book on medicine, setting forth its general and particular laws to the full extent necessary, and yet with apt brevity.

Volume I: General Medicine

My plan is to deal with the general aspects of each of the two divisions of medicine—the speculative and the practical. Then I shall treat of the general principles applicable to the diagnosis of the properties of the simples, following this with a detailed account of them. I shall, then, take up the disorders which befall each individual member, beginning with an account of its anatomy, and that of its auxiliary. The anatomy of the several members and their auxiliaries is dealt with in the first book. Having completed the account of the anatomy, I shall show how the health of the member is to be maintained.

This subject being completed, I proceed to a general discourse about general diseases: their causes, the signs by which they are recognized, and the modes of treatment. After this, I pass on to the special diseases and will point out in as many cases as possible: (1) the general diagnosis of their characters, causes and signs; (2) the special diagnostic features; (3) the general rules of treatment; (4) the special methods of treatment by (a) simples; and (b) compounded medicines.

I include specially designed tables under the subject of simples to enable you to survey the facts rapidly as to the adjuvants for treating disease by simples.

I have deemed it best to consider compounded medicines, their adjuvants, and how to mix them separately in a formulary. This it is my intention to compose after the special subjects are dealt with. Disorders not confined to one member are described in this book; cosmetics are spoken of, and the knowledge set forth in previous books is assumed. God helping me to complete this volume, the formulary will be added to it. Every follower of my teachings, who wishes to use them profitably, should memorize most of this work, even though he not understand it all.

It is my intention to prepare further volumes if God should prolong my life still further, and if circumstances prove propitious. [Avicenna was to complete five volumes of which this is the translation of the first volume. LB.]

...

A brief summary of the contents of remaining volumes, II, III, IV, and V of *The Canon* are: [Volumes I, II and V have been translated into English. LB]

Volume II: Simple Drugs

This volume gives a detailed material medical pharmacology and therapeutics of drugs. It has two parts.

Part One. General Principles: These deal with the temperament or constitution of drugs, and how it is determined: (1) by experiment; and (2) by deduction. Conditions of the experiment such as, its being on the human body, drug to be free of extrinsic and intrinsic alterations, the trial to be allopatric and made on simple diseases, drug to be qualitatively and quantitatively corresponding to the severity of the disease, etc., have been described. Part one also gives an account of all the actions which drugs may possess and describes the method of collection and preservation of the various herbal and other products.

Part Two. List of Drugs: It gives 797 drugs in seriatim according to the Abjad system. The properties of each drug have been described under the following headings: general description of the drug, tests for its purity, qualities, general and special actions on each system of the body or on special diseases; specific actions; antidotal properties; alternative remedies and adjuvants.

Volume III: Diseases of Individual Members

In Volume III, the various diseases have been discussed systematically, with their etiology, symptoms, diagnosis, prognosis and treatment with simple drugs. Special mention may be made of the following sections:

Head: brain, (intemperaments, headache in all its aspects, organic diseases of the brain, epilepsy, paralysis, etc.) eye, ear, nose, mouth, throat, and teeth. Chest: lungs, heart, breasts. Alimentary tract: stomach, intestines, liver, gall bladder and spleen. Intestines and the anus, disorders of the rectum. Urinary tract: the kidneys, bladder and urine. The male reproductive system; the female reproductive system, conception, pregnancy, and diseases of women. Muscles: joints, and feet.

Volume IV: General Diseases

Part One. Fevers: general description of fevers; their periodicity; causes such as constipation, diarrhea, dietetic indiscretion; excessive activity; excessive wakefulness; fear or anger; pain, inflammation, putrefaction, humoural disturbances; etc. Diagnosis of fevers; epidemic fevers; small pox; phthisis. Prognosis. Management of symptoms such as thirst, rigors, diarrhea, vomiting, sleeplessness, pain, headache, etc. Treatment of fevers: general and specific. Subject of crisis.

Part Two. Boils and swellings. Leprosy. Minor surgery. Wounds and their general treatment. Injuries: fractures and dislocations. Ulcers. Glandular swellings.

Part Three. Poisoning with mineral, vegetable and animal products. Bites from animals and man.

Part Four. Beauty culture. Leanness and obesity. Hair, nails and skin. Treatment of offensive odors and discolorations including leucoderma. Pediculosis. Pitting from small pox, etc.

Volume V: The Formulary

This volume gives details of special prescriptions and antidotes; their form such as pills, powders, syrups, decoctions, confections, elixirs, etc, and their method of preparation. A thorough discourse about laxatives; purgative and non-purgative powders; medicinal powders, dosages; electuaris; potions and thickened juices; jams and preserves; pills; greens and cereals; lotions; and ointments and dressings. Prescriptions for different diseases. Weights and measures.

Avicenna's Introduction
The Basis of Health and Disease and the Inevitability of Death

Medicine comprises two parts, one theoretical, and one practical, though both are really speculative science. That which is specially named theory relates to the formation of opinions and the showing of the evidence upon which they are based, without reference to the mode of acting upon them. Thus this part deals with the temperaments, the humours, the drives, and with the forms, the symptoms, and the causes of disease. That which is specially named practical relates to the mode of acting upon this knowledge, and the prescription of a regimen.

For instance, it is that part of medicine which helps us understand how the health of the body is to be maintained in this or that state, and by what means we can heal the diseases with which the body is afflicted. Practical does not refer to the performance of surgical operations. It is the art which teaches us in what way to procure healing— the healing art.

The human being takes its origin from two things: (1) the male semen, which plays the part of factor; and (2) the female menstrual discharge, which provides the matter.

Each of these is fluid and moist, but there is more wateriness and earthly substance in the female blood and female sperm, whereas air and fire are predominant in the male sperm. It is essential that at the outset of the congelation of the two components there should be moisture, even though earth and fire are found in the product. The earth provides the firmness and rigidity; the fire provides the maturative power. These give the coagulum (*"He created man from a clot"* Quran, 96:2) a certain hardness or firmness. But this hardness is not as great in degree as that possessed by a stone or glass. For these are either not soluble at all or only soluble to a degree imperceptible to our senses, however long one exposes them to solvents. Were the hardness comparable to this, the product of conception would never suffer injury however long or however persistently a solvent were applied. But that is not so. The act is contrary.

Our bodies are exposed to injury from two directions—externally and internally. The source of internal injury is the dissipation of the moisture from which we are created, and this dissipation proceeds in an orderly manner. The second source is the putrefactive breakdown and metamorphosis of the humour into a form such that the fermentative phenomena of life are no longer able to proceed.

The second source of injury differs from the first in that dryness is here introduced by virtue of depravity of humour; and this dryness continues neutralizing the moisture of the body until the form ceases to have a capacity for life.

Finally, the putrefactive breakdown disperses the vitality, because it first destroys the moisture and then disperses it, and simply dry ash is left behind.

Therefore we see that these two sources of destruction [of the living product of conception] are different from those arising from other causes —such as, freezing cold, torrid heat, grave forms of loss of continuity, various maladies. But it is in regard to the first two named sources of destruction that we find the more important factors relative to the question of the preservation of health.

Each of them takes its origin from extrinsic and intrinsic agents. The extrinsic agents are for example, the atmosphere, which is a solvent and putrefacient. The intrinsic agents are, for example, the innate heat, which is the agent within us through which moisture is dispersed: the extraneous heat generated within us from the aliments, and through other agents which cause putrefactive changes in the [native] moistures.

All these agents mutually aid one another in rendering the body dry. And yet it is true that our perfection and soundness and the power to perform our various actions depend on a degree of dryness of the blood. But the degree of dryness becomes relatively greater and greater until we die. Therefore, this dryness is inevitable.

If we were at the outset essentially composed of moisture, heat would have to overcome it or else the heat would be choked by it. Therefore the heat continues to exert its own effect, that is, it produces more and more desiccation. But whatever degree of dryness there might be at the outset (of life), it reaches equilibrium, and remains so until the limit of equilibrium in regard to dryness is reached. The heat remaining constant, the dryness is now relatively greater than before for the matter is less, and hence holds more.

Therefore it is not difficult to understand that the dryness passes on beyond the stage of equilibrium, and goes on steadily increasing until the whole of the moisture of the body is consumed. Therefore (we may say) that the innate heat is the cause of its own extinction, for it is itself the reason for its own matter being consumed. We may compare it to the flame of a lamp; the light goes out when all the matter has been used up.

As the dryness increases, the innate heat diminishes. The loss continues unceasingly till death, and the moisture which is lost is not restored. The loss goes on more and more.

The dryness (of the body) is increased in two ways: by lessening of the power of receiving matter; by lessening of the native moisture resulting from dispersal of the (innate) heat. The heat becomes more feeble because dryness predominates in the substance of the members, and because the innate moisture becomes relatively less. The innate moisture is to the innate heat as the oil of a lamp is to the flame. For there are two forms of moisture in the flame: water, which holds its own, and oil, which is used up. So, in a corresponding manner, the innate heat holds its own in respect of the innate moisture, but is used up *pari passu* with increase of extraneous heat, due, for example, to defective digestion, which is comparable with the aqueous moisture of the flame. As the dryness increases, the innate heat lessens, and the result is natural death.

For the reason why the (human) body does not live any longer than it does lies in the fact that the initial innate moisture holds out against being dispersed both by the alien heat and by the heat in the body itself (both that which is innate and that derived from bodily movement). And this resistance is maintained as long as the one is weaker than the other, and as long as something is provided to replace that which has been thus dispersed, to wit, from the aliment. Furthermore, as we have already stated, the power or drive which operates upon the aliment in order to render it useful in this way only does so up to the end of life.

Therefore, we may say that the art of maintaining health is not the art of averting death or of averting extraneous injuries from the body or of securing the utmost longevity possible to the human being. It is concerned with two other things: (1) the prevention of putrefactive breakdown; and (2) the safeguarding of innate moisture from too rapid dissipation and maintaining it at such a degree of strength that the original type of constitution peculiar to the person shall not change even up to the last moment of life.

This is secured by a suitable regimen, namely: (a) one which will ensure the replacement of the innate heat and moisture which are dispersed from the body as exactly as possible; and (b) a regimen which will prevent any agents which would lead to a rapid dessication from gaining the upper hand excluding agents which produce a normal desiccation; (c) one which safeguards the body from the development of putrefactive processes within it and from the influence of alien heat (whether extraneous or intrinsic) because all bodies have not the same degree of innate moisture and innate heat. There is a great diversity in regard to them.

Moreover, every person has his own term of life, during which the desiccation inevitable to his temperament (constitution) and the degree of innate heat, and of innate moisture can be withstood.

Nevertheless, factors may arise which assist desiccation, or are injurious in some other way. For which reason, many assert that the former are natural causes of death, whereas the latter are accidental. And under this view, the art of maintaining health consists in guiding the body to its natural span of life by paying attention to whatever things conduce thereto. There are two drives to be fostered by the doctor in striving for this object: (1) the nutritive drive whereby that is replaced which is constantly being lost to the body namely earthiness and aquosity; and (2) the sensitive drive (animal faculty), that is, the pulsatile faculty which is concerned with the replacement of that which is lost to the body by the breath namely air and fire. And since aliments are only potentially like the thing nourished, an alternative drive had to be created so that they could be changed actually into the likeness of the thing nourished. In this way the aliment becomes effective.

The instruments and channels necessary for this had to be created also—namely the means by which material is attracted, expelled, retained, and digested (sequence by sequence, turn by turn).

Therefore, we may say that the essential considerations in the art of preserving the health consist in maintaining equilibrium between all these various concomitant factors. But there are seven matters concerning which special care must be expended to ensure just proportion: (1) equilibrium of temperament; (2) selection of the articles of food and drink; (3) evacuation of effete matters; (4) safeguarding the composite; (5) maintaining the purity of the air respired; (6) guarding against extraneous contingencies; and (7) moderation in regard to the movements of the body and the motions of the mind, with which may be included sleep and wakefulness.

From all these considerations you will now perceive that there is no single fixed limit to which equilibrium or health is to be assigned. None of the temperaments enters into it. Health and equilibrium vary (in range) from time to time. That is to say, it is a state comprised—within two limits.

On Healthy Living: Exercising, Massaging, Bathing, Eating, Drinking, Sleeping and Treating Fatigue

1.1. A Word About Exercise

Since the regimen[1] for maintaining health consists essentially in the regulation of: (1) exercise; (2) food; and (3) sleep, we may begin our discourse with the subject of exercise. We may define exercise as voluntary movement entailing deep and hurried respiration.

Once we direct the attention towards regulating exercise as to amount and time, we shall find there is no need for such medicines as are ordinarily required for remedying diseases dependent on [abnormal] matters, or diseases of temperament consequent upon such. This is true provided the rest of the regimen is appropriate and proper

We know that this must be so when we reflect how in regard to nutriment, our health depends on the nutriment being appropriate for us and regulated in quantity and quality. For not one of the aliments which are capable of nourishing the body is converted into actual nutriment in its entirety. In every case digestion leaves something untouched, and nature takes care to have that evacuated. Nevertheless, the evacuation which nature accomplishes is not a complete one. Hence at the end of each digestion there is some superfluity left over. Should this be a frequent occurrence, repetition would lead to further aggregation until something measurable has accumulated. As a result, harmful effete substances would form and injure various parts of the body. When they undergo decomposition, putrefactive diseases arise [bacterial infections, Tr.]. Should they be strong in quality, they will give rise to an intemperament; and if they should increase in quantity, they would set up the symptoms of plethora which have already been described. Flowing to some member, they will result in an inflammatory mass, and their vapors will destroy the temperament of the substantial basis of the breath.

That is the reason why we must be careful to evacuate these substances. Their evacuation is usually not completely accomplished without the aid of toxic medicines, for these break up the nature of the effete substances. This can be achieved only by toxic agents, although the drinking of them is to a certain extent deleterious to our nature. As Hippocrates says: "Medicine purges and ages." More than this the discharge of superfluous humour entails the loss of a large part of the natural humidities and of the breath, which is the substance of life. And all this is at the expense of the strength of the principal and auxiliary members, and therefore they are weakened thereby. These and other things account for the difficulties incident to plethora, whether they remain behind in the body or are evacuated from it.

Now exercise is that agent which most surely prevents the accumulation of these matters, and prevents plethora. The other forms of regimen assist it. It is this exercise which renews and revives the innate heat, and imparts the necessary lightness to the body, for it causes the subtle heat to be increased and daily disperses whatever effete substances have accumulated; the movements of the body help to expel them conveying them to those parts of the body whence they can readily leave it. Hence the effete matters are not allowed to collect day after day and besides this, as we have just said, exercise causes the innate heat to flourish and keeps the joints and ligaments firm, so as to be always ready for service, and also free from injury. It renders the members able to receive the nutriment, in being free from accumulated effete matters. Hence it renders the attractive faculty active, resolves fibrosis in the tissues, rendering the members light and the humidities attenuated, and it dilates the pores of the skin.

To forsake exercise would often incur the risk of "hectic," because the instinctive drives of the members are impaired, inasmuch as the deprivation of movement prevents the access to them of the innate breath. And this last is the real instrument of life for every one of the members.

The value of exercise includes the following: (1) it hardens the organs and renders them fit for their functions; (2) it results in a better absorption of food, aids assimilation, and, by increasing the innate heat, improves nutrition; (3) it clears the pores of the skin; (4) it removes effete substances through the lungs; (5) it strengthens the physique. Vigorous exercise invigorates the muscular and nervous system.

1.1.1. The Varieties of Exercise

There are two main forms of exercise: (a) that pertaining to the ordinary human undertakings; and (b) that which is undertaken for its own sake—namely, for the advantage accruing from its pursuit. [i.e., sports, athletics, gymnastics, etc.]

There are differences between the two forms. One is strong and powerful, the other weak and light; one is speedy, the other slow. Athletics implies strenuous exertions combining swiftness with energy. Recreative exercise, undertaken for relaxation, implies leisurely movements. There are all grades between these extremes, and there is a mean between them [called moderate exercise]. List of the forms of exercise include:

1.1.2. Strenuous Exercises

Strenuous forms include wrestling contests; boxing; quick marching; running, jumping over an object higher than one foot; throwing the javelin; fencing; equitation or horsemanship [hunting: Galen, Rhazes].[2] Also, clapping the two hands alternately before and behind, with a quick motion while standing on tip-toes [dancing[3] (Oribasius), swimming (*ibid.*)]. These are special forms of individual athletic exercises.

1.1.3. Mild Exercises

The following are recreative or milder modes of exercise: swaying or swinging to and fro, as when being carried in a litter; standing or reclining in small boats; fishing; sailing; being driven in horse-carriages or carried on camels or in palanquins or a horse-litter.

1.1.4. Vigorous Exercises

Among the more vigorous exercises are those performed by soldiers in camp, in military sports; field running: where a man runs on the field from end to end to and fro, lessening the distance each time until finally he comes to a stand in the middle; combat with one's shadow; exercise with the leather bag [which is filled with flour or sand, and hung to the level of the person's navel]; long jumping; high jumping; playing with a large ball [inflated skins or leather]; playing with a small, wooden ball on horseback [i.e., polo]; playing with a small wooden ball on horseback [i.e., polo] are also included along with stone-throwing; lifting heavy stones or weights, either while standing, or carrying them; scaling ropes; running galloping horses round in a circle; [leaping with a weight on the shoulders which exercises the spine: Galen].

There are various forms of wrestling. For instance, in one form, one of the wrestlers grasps the other and holds him by the tips of the hands. The other tries to get loose from his opponent. In another, one wrestler grips the right hand of his opponent and takes the left hand with his left, the two facing one another; then the one raises the other up into the air, and turns him round sometimes in the bent position, sometimes in the upright position. Again, the two wrestlers may press against one another breast to breast or one holds the other by the neck to pull him to the ground. Or, one may twist and press with his feet, twisting his legs round his opponent, or turn heel to heel. Various other movements of that kind are in vogue among wrestlers.

1.1.5. Brisk Exercises

Exercises involving swiftness include interchanging places with a partner as swiftly as possible, each jumping to and fro, either in time [to music] or irregularly. Another exercise is carried out with two stakes. The man jumps backwards repeatedly without moving his position, and plunges the two stakes on either side, one pace apart, causing the one on the right to go to the left, and the one on the left to go to the right. This is to be done as swiftly as possible.

Exercises involving vigor and swiftness should alternate with mild exercises, or with rest. The manner of the exercises should also be diversified, so that they are not always performed in the same way.

1.1.6. The Instructions for Exercise

There is an exercise which is appropriate for each individual. Gentle exercise (i.e., swinging: rocking in a swing) is beneficial for those who are debilitated by fevers or who are convalescing and can neither walk nor sit—for those weakened by a draught of hellebore and the like or for those whose diaphragm has been rendered enfeebled by disease. When it is done gently, it tends to induce sleep, and disperse flatulence, relieves various disorders of the head (i.e., stupor, forgetfulness) provokes the appetite, and favors movement of the bowels.

To ride in a litter [horse, camel, palanquin, etc.] is appropriate for those afflicted with semitertian fever, composite fevers, phlegmatic fevers, those who are dropsical, or have gouty pains or renal disorder. For this form of exercise renders effete matter in a condition favorable for excretion, and may be made gentle for the feeble, more vigorous for the more vigorous. Greater movement is produced in the humours by riding in a carriage, but when doing so one should face backwards, because this is better when the eyesight is weak, and it is an advantage to have the shadow in one's face.

Boating and sailing: to go out in a small boat, or in a larger sailing vessel is beneficial for lepra, dropsy, apoplexy, dilatation of the stomach and coldness of the stomach. For if the person is near the shore he is incited to vomit, and then when that subsides, the stomach is benefited. But to go on the high seas is more efficient for clearing up such disorders as we have named, because the mind is diverted by successive gladness and misery, and the organs of nutrition receive benefit in proportion to the exercise of the body itself.

1.2. The Exercises for Special Organs of the Body

Each member should be exercised in a manner appropriate for itself. (1) The hands and feet—the proper way to exercise these is obvious. (2) The organs of respiration, and the muscles of the chest. These may be exercised in various ways: (a) By singing and "vociferation." The voice is sometimes deep, sometimes loud, sometimes abrupt, sometimes used in all modes in one exercise. By this means the condition of the mouth, uvula, lips, tongue is improved. The muscles of the neck are improved in appearance. The color of the skin is improved. The chest is expanded. (b) Exercises in which the expiration is forced and the breath is held. These benefit the whole body, because they open up and purify the channels, including those of the breath.[4]

However, to use a loud voice for a long time is injurious because by continuing it vigorously too much air is taken in, which is itself harmful, and by continuing it too long, air must be expelled unduly, and this also is harmful. Therefore the rule is to begin gently, by reading aloud, speaking more and more loudly up to a certain point and then allowing the voice to sink by degrees. If the time occupied in this exercise is moderate, it is very helpful, but if the time is too long, there is risk of injury to health.[5]

Vision is exercised by inspecting minute objects, and sometimes by arranging that they are only poorly illuminated.

Audition is exercised by listening to faint sounds, or sometimes to loud ones.

Exercises appropriate to each individual member will be referred to when we speak of the maintenance of the health of each organ in the special volume.

1.2.1. Important Instructions

Whatever the exercise, one must ensure that its vigor or heating effect is not likely to affect some weak organ directly. Such an organ should only bear the brunt of the exercise secondarily. For instance, a person with varicose veins should not use an exercise in which the feet are much used. He should substitute an exercise which employs the upper parts of the body the neck, the head, and the hands. In this way the brunt of the effect of the exercise is borne first by the upper parts and by the feet last.

The exercise must be modified if the person is debilitated. If he is robust it should be made vigorous. You realize now that every organ has its own peculiar form of exercise. That the exercise for the eye is to gaze upon something delicate; that the exercise to strengthen and expand the chest is vocal, and consists of graduated singing exercises. Similarly with the teeth and the ear. Every member is considered in this way in the chapter specially devoted to it.

1.2.2. The Time for Exercise

The time to choose for beginning exercise is when the body is free from impurities in the internal organs and blood vessels so that there is no risk of unhealthy chyme being dispersed through the body by the exercise. Yesterday's food should have passed both gastric and hepatic digestion, and also intravascular digestion—the time for the next meal now approaching, as can be ascertained by examining the urine as to its substance and color.

If it is some time before the next meal is due, and there is a need for more nutriment, and the urine shows igneity (i.e., is high-colored), the natural yellowness having now passed off, it indicates that exercise at this time would be detrimental, namely by exhausting the strength.

For this reason, some people say that when vigorous exercise has to be undertaken, it is best that the stomach should not be quite empty: that there should still be a little food, and that this should be substantial in winter and light in summer.

Moreover, it is better to choose a time for exercise when one is not hungry, and when one is hot and moist rather than cold and dry. But the best time is when the state is between the two. Exercise in a man of hot and dry temperament may lead to illness, and he will benefit by avoiding it at such a time.

It is necessary, then, for a person who is about to take exercise that he should first get rid of the effete matters of the body by way of the intestines and bladder. Should friction be used in preparation for exercise, with the object of helping the bowels and opening the pores of the skin, it should be carried out with a rough towel and be followed by inunction with sweet (perfumed) oil made warm by being held in the hollow of the palm. This inunction is done according to rule until the limbs show a florid blush; the massaging should not be too forcible nor the penetration too great. It is done with the hands, which pass over many various positions in order to ensure that every part of the muscular system has been dealt with. When completed, the massage is stopped and exercise may begin.

In the spring, the best time for exercise is round midday and it should be done in a moderately warm room. In summer, the exercise should be done earlier. In winter, it should be delayed until evening, but there are other objections to doing so. Consequently, in winter, the place used should be made moderately warm, to enable the exercise to be carried out at a time when the aliment is digested and the effete matters have been expelled.

1.3. The Amount of Exercise

Three things must be taken into consideration: (1) the color—as long as the skin goes on becoming florid, the exercise may be continued. After it ceases to do so, the exercise must be discontinued; (2) movement—exercise may be continued as long as the movement is moderated; (3) the condition of the organs-exercise must not be continued after they show any puffiness. Should the insensible perspiration lessen and the visible sweating stop, the exercise must stop. Should the action of the skin have ceased, one applies a strongly-diaphoretic oil as an inunction, especially if the exercise were one which exerted the breathing.

At the conclusion of the first day's exercise, you will know the degree of exercise allowable and when you know the amount of nourishment the person can bear, do not make any change in either on the second day. Arrange that the measure of aliment, and the amount of exercise shall not exceed the limit ascertained on the first day.

1.4. Massage

Varieties: (1) hard massage: this stretches and contracts, and braces the body; (2) soft massage has a relaxing effect; (3) repeated massage diminishes the fat of the body; (4) moderately hard massage; (5) rough massage: this is done with rough towels. It draws the blood rapidly to the surface; and (6) gentle massage is done with the palm or with soft towels. It draws the blood together and retains it in one member.

The object of friction is to render thin persons heavier, and heavy persons thinner; to brace flabby persons, and to modify those who are not pliable enough (giving tone to the body).

1.4.1. The Preparatory Massage

Massage as a preparatory to athletics. The massage begins gently, and then becomes more vigorous as the time approaches for the exercise.

1.4.2. Restorative Massage

Massage as a sequel to athletics is called restorative friction. This produces repose. Its object is to disperse the effete matter formed in the muscles and not expelled by the exercise. It causes them to disperse and so removes fatigue [the feeling of lassitude]. Such friction is soft and gentle, and is best done with oil [or perfumed ointments: Aeg.]. It must not be hard, or heavy, or rough, because that would roughen the members. Young men would be hindered in growth. But for adults it is less harmful.

It is less detrimental to err on the side of hardness than on that of softness, because it is easier to correct undue dispersal [of effete matters] than to prepare the tissues (by soft friction) for the reception of effete substances. On the other hand, hard and rough friction to an excess in youths is a hindrance to their growth.

You will learn about this under the heading of the proper time for massage. For the present it will suffice to say that restorative friction should be begun vigorously at first, and with oil; that then it should be moderated, but not stopped, until all roughness has gone. It is best that many persons should do it together. The person, having been rubbed, now stretches out his massaged limbs to help to expel the effete matters from them, and a broad bandage or binder is applied over the regions to which the muscles concerned belong. He should hold his breath as long as he can, while relaxing his abdominal muscles if he should at the same time make his thoracic muscles tense, if he can. Finally, he makes his abdominal muscles tense again. In this way the intestines are given a certain amount of restorative massage. One may pause to take a breath between the exercises; or sometimes restorative massage may be given in the middle of the exercise. Thus, it may be omitted or resorted to according to whether the exercise is to be prolonged or not. A person who desires restorative massage does not need much preliminary massage, unless there is something about his condition with which he is not satisfied. If he does not desire restorative massage he will undergo more thorough preliminary massage. If fatigue should be experienced, inunction with oil will be employed, as we have stated. If he should experience a sense of dryness, the massage will be increased until the natural mean condition is attained.

Causing friction without massage (compression) is beneficial if sleep is due, because it cheers the body and prevents humid matters from flowing into the joints.

1.5. Bathing and Bath Houses

For the type of person whose regimen we are discussing, a bath which induces resolution is not required, because his body is inwardly pure. A person does not need the bath except in order to derive a gentle warmth from it, and a moderate amount of moisture. That is why such persons should not stay long in it.

If such persons employ a full length (copper) bath, they should stay in it only until the color of the skin becomes red, and the skin becomes puffy; they should leave it as soon as dispersal (of humours) begins. The surrounding air should be moistened by a sweet-water spray The actual washing should now be quick and the bath left quickly.

A person should not go into the bath immediately after exercise. He should rest properly first.

The forms of bath have already been referred to and are dealt with again in another place.

At this point we should state that all who propose to bathe should pass through the successive rooms of the bath-house according to rule, and not linger in the hot room long enough to cause harm; they should stay long enough in the rest-room to give time for the dispersal of the effete substances, otherwise there is a risk of weakness which will interfere with digestion and leave a susceptibility to the causes of septic fevers.

A person who wishes to become stout should take his bath after a meal, if he is not likely to develop obstructions in consequence.

If he is of hot temperament, he may guard against the formation of obstructions by drinking oxymel [a mixture of vinegar and honey].

If he is of cold temperament, he should take penny-royal and capsicum.

If it is desired to reduce fat, and to procure the resolution of the humours, the person should bathe while fasting, and stay a long time in the bath.

1.5.1. The Beneficial Effects of Baths

The benefits are (1) induction of sleep; (2) dilation of pores; (3) cleansing of skin; (4) dispersal of the undesirable waste matters; (5) maturation of abscesses; (6) drawing of nutriment towards the surface of the body; (7) assistance to the physiological dispersion and excretion of poisonous matters; (8) prevention of diarrhea; and (9) removal of fatigue effects.

1.5.2. The Injurious Effects of Baths

To ensure against impairment of health the bather should wait till after the gastric and hepatic digestions are both completed. Where there is any risk of the bilious humour undergoing fermentative decomposition, and one wishes to bathe fasting, the aliment should be attenuant. But a person of hot temperament, in whom the bilious humour is plentiful, should not enter the hot chamber at all. The best things for such persons to take are: bread soaked with the juice of fruits or rose-water. Cold drinks should not be taken either while in the bath or when leaving it, for the pores are now open, and coldness would speedily enter and pass towards the principal organs and damage their functional capacity. Articles which are, very heating (hot) should also be avoided, especially water because thereby there is a risk of the warmth penetrating rapidly to the principal organs and this predisposes to wasting and hectic. Further, such persons should take care not to leave the bath suddenly, or to uncover the head, thus exposing the body to cold. If it is winter, the body should be well covered with towels.

A person suffering from fever should avoid the bath at the febrile period. The same applies to a person suffering from any form of loss of continuity, or from inflammation.

From the above, therefore, it will be clear to you that baths have the following effects: warming, cooling, humectant, desiccants beneficial, harmful.

Injurious effects include the fact that the heart is weakened if the person stay too long in the bath. The bath produces syncope and nausea, sets stagnant humours in circulation, disposes them to undergo putrescence, and to pass down into the weaker members, with consequent inflammatory deposits in both internal and external members.

1.5.3. Bathing in Cold Water and Starting With It

The bath is only beneficial if all the proper rules are observed, and if the age of the person, his physique and build, are suitable, and the seasons is appropriate (i.e. the summer). The contra indications are: nausea, or a feeling of satiety associated with indigestion; vomiting; or diarrhea; or want of sleep; or nasal catarrh. The person must not be at the age of boyhood, nor at old age. [Therefore he must be in the prime of life.] The moment chosen for the bath should be one at which the body is light and the movements appropriate.

The object of bathing with cold water following upon one with hot water is to make the external parts stronger and to retain the natural heat. For this purpose the water used should not be very cold, but of a medium temperature.

Bathing with cold water after exercise. Here the preparatory massage should be more vigorous than usual. The customary inunction with oil is employed as well before the exercise, which must be less vigorous than usual. The exercise completed, the person plunges into the cold water tank, so as to harden all the members at once. He stays in the cold water in proportion to his lightness, and as long as he can without shivering ensuing. Then, having come out of the water, let him be rubbed as we have described (i.e. till the skin is red) and let him take more food than drink. The time which elapses before the natural color returns to the skin must be noted, because if the color returns rapidly, the duration of the cold bath was reasonable, whereas if there is delay, it shows that the stay in the water was too prolonged. In this way the person will know the proper duration of the bath for the future.

Should the person wish to reenter the water after the massage, and after regaining his color and normal heat, he must on this occasion enter the water gradually, and on a hot summer's day before the hottest part of the day, and when no wind is blowing. He must not do so when in a state of lassitude after coitus, or after a meal which has not had time to digest, or after emesis, or after evacuation of the bowels or after gastro-enteritis, or insomnia, or if the body or stomach be enfeebled.

Cold bathing should not be done after exercise except in the case of the very robust. Even then the rules which we have given should be followed. To use cold baths in the ways we have named drives the natural heat suddenly into the interior parts, and then invigorates the strength so that the person should leave the bath twice as strong as when he entered.

1.6. Concerning Food

In seeking to maintain health care must be taken that the essential basis of the meal is not in medicinal nutrients like potherbs, fruits, and such-like. For things which are tenuous in character over oxidize the blood, while those which are dense render the blood phlegmatic and the body heavy.

1.6.1. Menu

The meal should include: (1) meat especially kid of goats; veal, and year-old lamb; (2) wheat, which is cleaned of extraneous matter and gathered during a healthy harvest without ever having been exposed to injurious influences; (3) sweets of appropriate temperament; (4) fragrant wine of good quality.

Any other kinds of food can only be regarded as a sort of medicament or preservative.

The more nutritious fruits are: figs, grapes (ripe and sweet), dates from countries and regions in which they are indigenous. But if superfluity arises after partaking of these fruits, speedy evacuation should be procured.

1.6.2. The Appetite

A person should not eat unless hungry. Nor should he delay his meal until the appetite has passed off. This rule does not apply in the case of the fictitious appetite met with in drunkards or the subjects of nausea. If fasting be continued the stomach will fill up with putrescent humours.

1.6.3. Hot Meals

In winter the food should be hot; in summer cold or only slightly warm. A food should not be served either hot or cold if it is likely to be spoiled thereby.

1.6.4. The Quantity of Food

Nothing is worse than to eat to repletion during a time of plenty after having been in a state of starvation during a time of famine, and vice versa. But the transition period is the worse. For we often see many people who lack food at a time of famine, and eat to repletion when a fertile year comes with fatal result. Great repletion is very dangerous in any case, whether in regard to food or to drink. For how often do not people over-eat, and perish from the consequent choking of the channels of the body?

1.6.5. The Order of the Meals

An error in eating or drinking any of the medicinal nutrients is to be corrected according to the digestion and maturation thereof. The person must be protected from the intemperament which is likely to arise. To effect this, one takes the contrary substance until the digestion is completed. Thus, if the aliment was cold (i.e., cucumber, gourd), temper it with its opposite (i.e., onions, leek). If the aliment was hot, temper it with the opposite (i.e., cucumber, purslane). If the aliment is binding, take some food which will open and evacuate, and then fast for a suitable period. A person in this state—and this is true for all who wish to maintain their health—should not partake of food until there is a definite appetite, and unless the stomach and upper small intestine have emptied themselves of the previous meal, because there is nothing more harmful to the body than to super impose digestive matter upon incompletely digested food. There is also nothing worse than nauseative indigestion especially when this is the result of bad foods. If these are gross, the following symptoms and illnesses arise: pains in the joints, in the kidneys; dyspnea, podagra, indurative enlargement of the spleen and liver, illnesses in which the serous or atrabilious humours are concerned.

If the foods were attenuated, then acute fevers, malignant fevers, and grave acute inflammatory disturbances would develop.

1.6.6. Aids to Digestion

However, it is sometimes really necessary to give a food or a substance like food, on the top of another food, by way of medicine. For example, if one has taken sharp and salty nutrients, one may further take humectant aliments which have no flavor, before the former have digested completely The chyme by which the body is nourished is then rectified. This is a suitable measure for cases of this kind, and the use of exercise is not indicated. The contrary holds good in the case of those who partake of gross foodstuffs and afterwards admix with them something which is speedily digested and acrid in taste.

1.6.7. Food and Exercise

A small amount of movement or activity after a meal allows the food to descend to the fundus of the stomach, especially if after this there is a desire to sleep. Mental excitement, emotion or vigorous exercise hinder digestion.

1.6.8. Seasons and Food

In winter, feebly nutrient foods like pot-herbs are not to be eaten. The aliments should be stronger and more solid in texture such as cereals, legumes, and the like. In summer, the contrary is true.

1.6.9. The Size of Meals

In regard to the quantity of food taken at a meal, no meal should be bulky enough to completely satisfy the appetite, One should rise from the table while some appetite or desire for food is still present for such remnants of hunger will disappear in the course of an hour. Custom is to be regarded in this regard, for a meal is injurious when it brings heaviness to the stomach, and wine is injurious when it exceeds moderation, and swims in the stomach.

If one ate to excess one day, one should fast the next, and a longer sleep should be taken in some place which is neither hot nor cold. If sleep refuses to come, one should take gentle walking exercise and allow neither rest nor recumbent position. A little pure wine should be taken. Rufus say: "Walking after a meal is gratifying to me, for it gives a good preparation for the evening meal."

1.6.10. Food and Sleep

A short sleep after a meal is useful; one should lie first on the right side, then on the left, and finally turn back again to the right side. If the body be covered with a number of wraps and the neck be raised, this will aid digestion. The limbs should slope downward and not upwards.

The standard size of the meal depends on usage and vigor. A normally robust person should take as much as will not produce a sense of heaviness, or a sense of tightness of the hypochondria. There should be no subsequent rumbling in the stomach or splashing of the food on bodily movement. Nausea should not be experienced, nor a canine appetite, nor loss of appetite, nor great disinclination for exertion, nor sleeplessness. The taste of the food should not repeat in the eructations. If the taste of food lingers in the mouth a very long time after the meal it shows that the latter was too heavy.

1.6.11. The Quantity of Food

Indications that the meal was moderate: the pulse does not become full; the breathing does not become shallow. The latter only occurs if the stomach is compressing the diaphragm, thus making breathing shallow and short. The pressure to be met by the heart increases after a large meal, and as the force of the heart does not diminish, the pulse becomes large and full.

1.6.12. Food and Temperament

The following should be observed: a person who experiences a sense of heat and flushing after a meal should not take a whole meal at one sitting, but partake of the food in small portions at short intervals to avoid the effects of repletion such as shivering followed by a sense of heat like that in a sthenic fever. This is due to the heating effect of the food; a person who cannot digest the amount of food appropriate for him should increase the number of articles of diet, but diminish the quantity; a person of atrabilious constitution needs a diet which is very humectant but not very heating; a person of choleric constitution needs a diet which is humectant and infrigidant; a person who generates hot inflammable blood needs feebly nutritious articles of food, which are cold. One who generates phlegmatic blood needs feebly nutritious articles of diet which are hot and attenuant.

1.6.13. The Order of the Dishes

The order in which the components of a meal are to be taken—a person who is desirous of maintaining his health needs to be watchful of this matter. Thus, one should not take a tenuous food, which is rapidly digested, after taking a very nutritious dish which is slowly digested. An exception to this rule has been named above. The reason is that the first article of food will be digested first and therefore float over the other, unable to enter the blood. Consequently it ferments and decomposes, and in addition sets up decomposition of the food next taken. The reverse order, therefore, is the one to adopt, so that the labile food will pass on with the other into the intestine, and then undergo complete digestion.

Fish and similar articles of food should not be taken after laborious work or exercise, because they undergo decomposition and then decompose the humours.

Some persons may be allowed to eat an article of food in which there is a styptic property as a preparatory to the actual meal.

1.6.14. The Prescription of the Diet

Some persons have an idiosyncrasy of the stomach in which the foods leave it very rapidly and do not stay in it long enough to undergo gastric digestion. This explains the necessity for taking the idiosyncrasy of the stomach and its temperament into consideration [along with other factors when drawing up a diet].

There are some persons in whom tenuous food, instead of being digested quickly as it should, undergoes decomposition in the stomach, whereas less rapidly digestible foods are digested more readily. The stomach of such a person is designated igneous. But other persons are exactly the opposite. Therefore the rules to be given must be adapted to the peculiarity of each patient.

The countries in which people live have also their own natural properties, which are distinct from the ordinary rule. This must also be borne in mind, and a test must be made to ascertain what the rule should be. Thus, a food which is often used, though injurious to a certain degree, may be more appropriate for a given individual than a food which he does not often take, though its character is good.

Then again, there is a food which is to be regarded as appropriate to everyone's physique and temperament. To change from such a diet would prove injurious and detrimental to him. Good and laudable foods may be injurious to some. They should therefore avoid them. But persons who are able to digest a bad foods should not be deceived, because (for all they know) they will some day give rise to bad humours and the consequent obstinate ailments.

Good food may often be allowed liberally in the case of persons in whom the humours are unhealthy, so long as diarrhea from intestinal weakness does not supervene in consequence. But if the person be of spare habit, and liable to have the motions loose, the diet should consist of moist aliments, because they are digested quickly, even though it is a fact that such persons can tolerate various heavy foods, and are less liable to be affected adversely by intrinsic noxae, and are more susceptible to the antagonistic influence of extraneous noxae.

1.6.15. The Excess of Meat

An active person accustomed to take much meat needs frequent bleeding. A person inclined to be frigid in temperament should drink substances which cleanse the stomach, intestines and the (mesenteric) veins including confections of spices and myrobalan electuary.

It is a bad practice to combine nutrients of diverse character in one meal and so prolong it. For by the time the last portion has entered the stomach, the first portion is already digested, and therefore the various contents of the stomach are not all at then same stage of digestion.

Palatability—one should remember too that aliment is best which has the most agreeable flavor for the walls of the stomach and the retentive faculty jointly apply themselves better to a food of good substance and the efficiency of the retentive power is assisted when the principal members all mutually concur the temperament of one being not more divergent from that of another than natural. That is the requisite condition. The conditions are not fulfilled, for instance, if the temperaments are not normal, or alike in the respective members. Thus, the temperament of the liver may differ to an unnatural extent from that of the stomach. Among noxious influences arising from the taste of aliments is that if very gross aliments are tasty, a person may be tempted to eat too freely of them.

1.6.16. The Number of Meals

In taking successive satiating meals, it is best for a person to take only one on one day and two on the next (morning and evening). But one must not be too strict in this rule, for if a person is accustomed to have two meals a day, and then takes only one, he will be weakened and his digestive faculty will suffer. A person of weak digestion should take two meals a day lessening the amount partaken. On occasion he may eat once a day. A person who is accustomed to take one good meal a day will, on resuming the habit of two meals a day, suffer from weakness, lack of energy, slackness. If he should take no food at bedtime, he will feel weak; and if he should take a late meal he will not be able to digest it, and will have acid eructations, nausea, bitter taste in the mouth, loose bowels and become moody, or irritable. This is because he has put into the stomach something to which it is not accustomed, and so he is liable to show some of the symptoms which befall a person whose aliment is not fully digested and these you are now acquainted with.

Among the symptoms arising when a person does not take a late meal are: subjective sensations at the cardiac orifice of the stomach, gnawing pains, a sensation of a void in the stomach so that all the interior organs and intestines feel as if they were suspended and, therefore, all clumped together. He passes scalding urine, and the feces produce a burning sensation as they are passed. There may be a feeling of cold in the extremities owing to the bilious humour being poured out into the stomach and irritating it and making it congested. This is more likely in persons of bilious temperament, and in those who have bilious humour in the stomach but not to an undue extent in the rest of the body; these suffer from loss of sleep, and keep turning over from one side to the other [in bed].

Persons then in whom the bilious humour is apt to accumulate in the stomach should take their meals divided, thereby taking the food quickly; the meal is taken before bathing. In other persons, exercise should be taken first, then the bath, and then the meal. The meal should not precede the bath in these cases. If circumstances demand that the meal betaken before the exercise, the food should consist of bread only, and to an amount no greater than can be easily digested. As it is necessary that the exercise should not be gentle if taken before food, so it is necessary that the exercise should be mild and gentle if it is taken after the meal.

When the appetite is depraved so that it prefers sharp tasting things to sweet or unctuous things, nothing is better than to procure emesis with such as oxymel with radish after fish.

A person who is stout should not eat at once after a bath, but should wait and take a little nap. He is best advised to take only one meal a day.

1.7. The Rules to be Observed After Meals

1.7.1. Exercise

One should not go to sleep immediately after a meal with the food still swimming in the stomach, and one should, as much as possible, abstain from much exercise after a meal, lest the food pass into the blood before it is sufficiently digested, or glide out of the stomach without being digested at all, or undergoes decomposition, since the exercise disturbs the gastric temperament.

1.7.2. Water and Meals

Nor should much water be drunk after a meal, for it causes the food to leave the coats of the stomach and float about. One should wait, and not drink fluids until the food has left the stomach which is evidenced by the sensation of lightness in the upper part of the abdomen. However, if there were urgent thirst one may take a modicum of cold water through a straw, and the colder it is the less one will require. Such an amount would soothe the stomach and keep the food together.

To sum up if a person must drink, it is better only to take so small an amount at the end of the meal (not during the meal), as will spread over and moisten the food, and therefore not be injurious.

1.7.3. Hunger

To go to sleep while thirsty is beneficial to cold and moist temperaments, but is injurious to those in whom the temperament is too warm, because of the bilious humour being too plentiful. The same is true as regards going to sleep while fasting.

Bilious humour comes to predominate in persons who fast and therefore flows into the stomach. Therefore when they eat any food it decomposes, and the same symptoms occur in them, whether asleep or awake, as when food corrupts. And, further more, there is loss of desire for food.

When there is loss of appetite for food something needs to be given to counteract this and relax the bowels. For this purpose something mild, like prune, should be given, or something which does not suggest nausea, like a laxative fruit juice (manna). Meals may be resumed after the appetite has returned. Those whose tissues are moist in virtue of natural humidity are liable to speedy aperierat action, and are in consequence not able to fast as long as those whose tissues are dry in virtue of only a small (degree of natural) humidity: unless the latter should by rich in humidities other than those inherent to the substance of the tissues, for these are proper, good and receptive, and in consequence the natural faculty is able to change them completely into (true) nutriment.

1.7.4. Beverages

To take wine after a meal is very unsatisfactory, for it is rapidly digested and enters the blood quickly and carries food on into the blood before it is properly digested. Obstructions and decompositions in this imperfectly digested aliment ultimately arise.

1.7.5. Sweets

Sweet things readily produce obstructions in the channels of the body because the attractive faculty-draws them into the blood before they have been properly digested. Obstructions culminate in various diseases of which dropsy is one.

1.7.6. Contamination of Food

Heaviness of the air or water, especially that of summertime, favors the decomposition of food. In this case, then, it is not harmful to take a tempered wine after a meal, or hot water in which xylaloes and mastic have been toiled.

1.7.7. Excessive Heat in the Stomach

If a person whose alimentary tract is hot and strong eats heavy food, it will give rise to flatulence in the stomach and fermentative ailments.

When a person takes a tenuous article of food upon an empty stomach, the latter contracts on it, and if he then takes something heavy, the stomach abandons the tenuous food and ceases digesting it, and it undergoes putrescence in consequence. This would be avoided by allowing an interval of time to elapse between the two kinds of food. Under these circumstances it is best to take the heavy food slowly, because then the hold which the stomach has on the tenuous food is not broken.

1.7.8. Dyspepsia

When a state of over repletion exists in regard to some meal, whether as a result of exercise (which causes undue hunger), or because a draught has been taken as well, then there will be a need for rapid emesis. If this should fail, or one cannot vomit, the person should sip hot water until the repletion is displaced and sleep supervenes. The person should therefore lie down to sleep. Let him sleep as long as he will. But should this not suffice, or should he be unable to go to sleep, reflect whether the natural course of events is likely to save you from procuring emesis. If so, good. If not, assist the natural power by any gentle laxative, such as myrobalan electuary, confection of roses, or origanum prepared with sugar or honey; or by the use of such things as cumin, spiced candies, asphodel and cabbage ptisan. It is not as bad to be replated with wine as with solid food.

Among the (aperient) remedies which are suitable after food are: aloes to the bulk of three chick-peas; or half a drachm of aloes, half a drachm of mastic, and a sixth of a drachm of niter.

Mild remedies are: turpentine resin to the amount of two or three chickpeas; niter in an equal quantity, or less, if necessary. Another much praised remedy is to use an epitheme with wine.

If none of these remedies succeed, let the patient sleep for a long time, and abstain from food for a whole day. Then, if he feels better, let him bathe, and place a hot blanket over the abdomen, and see that the aliments are tenuous.

1.7.9. Fullness of the Stomach

If the food is still not properly digested, in spite of all these measures, and heaviness, distension, and lack of energy are experienced, you may know that the veins are already overcharged with effete matters. Bulky and unneeded nutriment, even were it digested in the stomach, would hardly undergo the proper changes in the veins, and so would remain "crude" within them, and stretch them, even to bursting point. This is the explanation of the lack of energy, the heaviness, the desire to stretch oneself and the yawnings. The treatment in such a case consists in securing the release of the superfluities from the blood vessels.

If these are not the symptoms, but there is only a transient weariness, followed later by another form of weariness, this should be treated in the manner to be described.

1.7.10. Age and Diet

If a person should be very advanced in years, and his body does not derive as much benefit from the food as it did when he was young, and if his aliments become simply effete matters, then he should not eat as much as he used to do.

If a person is accustomed to a heavy diet and then lightens it by the use of attenuant foods, the new food material is unable to keep the channels of the body as full as bearer on resuming the heavy-foods, obstructions are brought about.

1.7.11. Ill Effects of Food

The injurious effects of heating or calefacient foods can be corrected by the use of syrup containing acetic acid, especially when made with seeds, for then the syrup is more efficient. If honey is used however, the simple syrup will suffice. The injurious effect of "cold" foods is corrected by the use of hydromel, and its syrup, and caraway.

Heavy and light foods—to correct aliments which are heavy, a person having a hot temperament should use acetous syrup made of strong seeds; a person with a cold temperament should use a little capsicum or peppermint.

Tenuous foods are better for the health, but less valuable for the vegetative faculties and strength. Heavy foods have the opposite value. Hence, for a person in need of a tonic, aliments which make strong chyme are necessary and-such as antagonize the hunger-feeling. But they should not be taken in greater quantity than can be digested. Heavy foods are better borne by those who take plenty of exercise or are accustomed to heavy work. Probably the deep sleep which this favors helps the digestion. But on the other hand they lose much by sweating. And as their livers seize whatever of the aliment has not yet digested fully, this paves the way for fatal illnesses towards the end of life, or at the beginning of life, the more so because they trust in their digestive powers too much. This power is really due to the deep sleep which is customary, and that is lost by old age.

1.7.12. Fruits

Fresh fruit is only good for those who carry out hard work, or take much exercise, or for persons with plenty of bilious humour, or during the height of summer. Fruit should be taken before a meal, namely, for instance, apricots, mulberries, melons, peaches, and prunes. But it is better to regulate oneself by using other articles of food than these, for they render the blood too watery, and so it is apt to ferment.

Hence the juices of fruits, unless taken at a seasonable time, pave the way for putrefactive processes. So, too, any food which comes to burden the blood with "crude" humour has this effect, though it is true that sometimes such a food may be beneficial. That is why people who make use of such aliments, even though they are primarily infrigidant, are likely to develop febrile diseases.

You will also realize that it is when watery humour is not dispersed, but lingers in the blood-vessels, that it usually becomes toxic. However, when exercise is taken before such aquosities have become aggregated, and exercise is taken immediately after eating the fruit, these aquosities will disperse and the noxious effect of the fruits is thereby lessened.

Note too that the presence of a crude serous humour or of wateriness in the blood prevents the nutrient part of the food from adhering to the tissues, some of the nutritive value of the food being lost as a consequence.

A person who partakes of fruit must (therefore) take walking exercise afterwards, and then eat something which will cause the (aquosities) to flow out.

1.7.13. Vegetables

Aliments which give rise to (1) wateriness; (2) crude, raw, immature humour and (3) gross humour and bilious humour, give rise to febrile diseases. This is because: (1) the watery parts permit putrescence to occur in the blood; (2) viscous gross substances close the orifices (of the juice-canals); and (3) the increase of bilious humour adds to the heat of the body, and renders the blood sharp.

Bitter pot-herbs are sometimes very advantageous in winter time, just as tasteless herbs are beneficial in summer time.

Correctives of unwholesome foods—if a person is bound to partake of unwholesome aliments, he should do so seldom and sparingly, and should counteract their action by combining with them something of a contrary effect. Thus, if a certain sweet food is injurious, he may counteract it by a sour aliment like vinegar, and pomegranate, and an acetous syrup prepared with sour wine and quince and the like, and also by procuring evacuation. Should it be a sour aliment that is injurious to him, he may follow it up with honey, or old wine, taking this before the maturation and digestion of the former are complete. If it be an oily aliment that is injurious, this can be corrected by (a) pungent articles, like chestnut, myrtle-seeds carob bean of Syria, the fruit of the lote tree, medlar; (b) bitters, such as conserved elecampane; (c) salt and sharp substances, such as capers, onions, garlic [that is, articles usually belonging to the second course of a meal], and other contraries.

If the body is in a state of repletion by unhealthy humours, this state may be counteracted by a liberal allowance of commendable attenuant aliments. If the body is one which is easily purged, moist and easily digested food should be made use of.

Galen says that a humid article of food is nutrient when it is separated from all other qualities, and is as it were tasteless-being neither sweet nor sour, bitter nor acrid, pungent nor salty.

A heavy food which is divided up into small portions will be better borne than one which is taken solid.

If dry aliments be taken plentifully, the strength will fail and the color will fade, and the nature become dry.

Fatty food produces lack of energy and vim, and creates a false appetite. Cold food produces lack of vim and is infrigidative (or attenuant). Sour food has the same effect as old age; it dries the body and makes it lean. Sharp and salty food is injurious to the stomach. Salty food is bad for the eyesight.

If an appropriate aliment is oily, and is followed by an uncommendable aliment, the latter will decompose it.

Viscous aliment experiences delay in passing through the intestine.

Citrul [a species of cucumber] passes down the intestine more rapidly if the rind is taken, as well, than if first peeled. Bread also passes down more quickly if the crust be taken as well than if it be deprived thereof by crumbling it through a sieve.

If a fatigued person, who is accustomed to a mild regimen should take heavy foods as for instance, a dish of rice with soured milk after a long fast, it will come about that his blood becomes sharp in quality and as if ebullient. Hence reducing his regimen would be indicated (e.g., blood-letting), though only to a moderate extent. A similar remedy is applicable when a person is angry. (Quick-tempered, the bilious humour easily becomes dominant or astir).

Note, too, that sweet aliment accelerates the nature before the food is matured and digested, and the blood is tainted in consequence.

1.8. Dietetic Aphorisms

Certain rules must be noted in regard to combining various articles of food. Indian observers and others have long taught that (1) milk must not be taken with sour foods; (2) fish must not be taken with milk for in that case chronic ailments such as leprosy[6] may develop; (3) pulse must not be taken with cheese or radishes or with the meat of flying birds; (4) a polenta[7] of barley-meal should not follow on a dish of rice made with soured milk;[8] (5) eatables should not have oil added, or oil which has stood in a brass vessel; (6) meat should not be taken when it has been roasted over live coals (with certain herbs).

To have several courses to a meal is injurious for two reasons: (1) the rate of digestion is diverse, for the part that digests more speedily is admixed with a part which is not yet digested; (2) a person may eat too much of one dish. Already in ancient times, too, persons who had been exercising themselves avoided this error, being satisfied to partake of meat alone in the morning, and bread alone at supper-time.

During the summer it is best to take the main meal at an hour when the temperature is cooler.

During a period of fasting the stomach sometimes fills with unhealthy humours.

Note further that when meat is roasted, and taken with onions and eggs [a special recipe *kabab*],[9] it is very nutritious; but it is slow in passing through the intestines, and lingers in the caecum. White soup [a Syrian dish containing rice, honey, onions] is nourishing, and when onion is added it dispels flatulencies; if onions are omitted, borborygmi arises.

Some people consider that grapes are good to take after roasted meats; but the contrary is really the case; they are very bad indeed. So too, is a dish containing dates, figs, and the like. But (dry) pomegranate seeds are good.

Fowl—the flesh of partridge is dry and constipating; but that of chicken is moist and relaxing to the bowels. Roast fowls are better if they have been prepared (stuffed) in the belly of a kid or lamb because that preserves their moisture. Chicken-broth tempers the humours strongly; more so than fowl-broth, though the latter is more nutritious.

Kid of goat is better when cold than when warm because the steam quiesces it. The flesh of lamb is better when hot because its unsatisfactory odor is thereby dispersed.

Meat boiled in water and vinegar [a Persian dish] should be served hot, and then needs no saffron in it. But if served cold saffron must be introduced.

Honey confections may be made with dates or wheat flour (sweetmeats); but they are unhealthy because they cause obstructions and evoke thirst.

Bread is an unsatisfactory food when it does not digest, more so than meat when it does not digest.

1.9. Concerning Water and Beverages

1.9.1. Water

Water is more suitable for attempered constitutions when it is moderately cold, than when it has been cooled by the addition of snow, especially if the snow were not pure. Even with good snow, there remains the objection that that which passes out from it is harmful to the nerves and the organs of respiration and all the internal organs. Moreover a person cannot tolerate it unless he is very full-blooded, and it will do harm sooner or later, even after the lapse of years.

Certain empirics assert that one must not mingle well-water with river-water, except by taking the one after the other has passed out of the stomach.

We have already spoken about the properties and choice of waters and how to correct them when bad. Addition with vinegar rectifies unhealthy waters.

One should remember that it is very harmful to drink water while fasting, or after exercise, or after the bath, especially when either of these was carried out on an empty stomach. It is also harmful to gratify the false thirst of the night, like that from which drunkards or topers suffer, or when the vegetative power strives to accomplish digestion in the face of a preceding satiety with water. If the thirst be very urgent, the water should be such as has been exposed to cool air, and rinse out the mouth with cold water. If this is not effective, some water may be taken out of a vessel with a narrow mouth. This is sometimes agreeable to a toper, who would not be hurt by drinking while fasting. If a person cannot avoid drinking while fasting, let him take water; especially if he has been taking exercise. In this case, let him first drink wine diluted with hot water.

False thirst is relieved by going to sleep without quenching it with fluid. For during sleep the natural power disperses the matter which is the cause of the thirst, and it does this more effectively if the thirst was not yielded to by a draught. To attempt to allay false thirst by a draught is to interrupt the digestive power, and the false thirst will return later because the humour giving rise to it is still there. When there is false thirst, water should not be taken rapidly and greedily, but through a straw.

It is bad to drink much cold water. If it is very imperative to do so, defer it till after a sufficient meal. Tepid water evokes nausea. Water warmer than that, if drunk frequently, weakens the [tone of the stomach. But when taken infrequently, it washes out the stomach and opens the bowels.

1.9.2. Beverages

White light wine is best for those who are in a heated state, for it does not cause headache. But sometimes it is humectant. It may relieve a headache when that is due to heat in the stomach.

Instead of a light white wine, one may use a wine which has been clarified by infusing honey or bread in it, especially if this is done two hours before the wine is required.

Heavy wine, if it is sweet, is best for a person who wants to put on weight and become strong. But he must beware of developing obstructions. Old red wine is best for a person of cold phlegmatic constitution. It is bad to drink wine after any of the various dishes, for the reason we have already explained. It should not be taken until after digestion, the food having passed into the small intestine. To drink wine upon food forming bad chyme, either during the meal or before it has digested, is bad because it causes the bad chyme to be absorbed and pass into the remote parts of the body. The same is true if wine is taken after fruit, especially melons.

It is better to begin with a small amount than a large one. To take two or even three glassfuls upon a meal is not hurtful to anyone accustomed thereto, or to a healthy person who has been bled.

Wine is beneficial for persons with a predominance of bilious humour, because it gets rid of the excess of this by provoking the urine. It is good for persons of humid temperament because it brings humidities to maturity. The better its aroma (bouquet) and taste, the more beneficial.

Wine is also very efficient in causing the products of digestion to become disseminated through the body. It cuts phlegm and disperses it. It separates of the bilious humour and draws it on into the urine. It renders the atrabilious humours more mobile and able to leave the system. It counteracts the harmful influence of this atrabilious humour by contrariety, and it breaks up all entanglements without the necessity of extraneous heat. The varieties of wine have been already enumerated in the proper place.

Wine does not readily inebriate a person of vigorous brain, for the brain is then not susceptible to ascending harmful gaseous products nor does it take up heat from the wine to any degree beyond what is expedient. Therefore it renders his mental power clearer than before; other talents are not affected in such an advantageous manner. The effect is different on persons who are not of this calibre.

A person who is weak in the chest, to the extent that wintertime is trying to the breathing, cannot [wisely] take much wine.

A person who wishes to take much wine should avoid taking much food beforehand, and the components of the meal should include diuretics. If he should become replete with food or wine, he should procure emesis and take hydromel (honey and water); then procure emesis again; then wash out the mouth with vinegar and honey, and apply cold water on the face.

If wine has an injurious effect on the body and is heating to the liver, the diet should include some dish containing for instance the juice of (sour) unripe grapes, and the like, and the articles of food which are generally served with the wine after the end of a meal (dessert) should include such as pomegranate, and tart things like citron.

If the wine is liable to go to the head, one should take less and take it dilute and clarified. After the meal, he should take such as quince with his wine.

If the harmful effect of wine consists in being heating to the stomach, the dessert should include toasted myrtle seeds and one should suck a few camphor lozenges and other astringent and acrid things.[10]

As you know, old wine is like a medicine. It is only feebly nutritious. New wine clogs the liver and produces a hepatic dysentery by giving rise to much gas. The best wine to take is that which is clear, white, tending to a red tinge, of good bouquet, and neither tart nor sweet in taste, neither old nor new.

A good drink which is widely known is made as follows: take three parts of marjoram, and one of water. Mix well. Boil to a fourth.

If a gnawing feeling come on after taking wine, take pomegranate, cold water and syrup of absinthe next morning. Enter the bath after partaking of a small meal.

Wine which is thoroughly diluted softens the stomach, makes it humid and allays thirst. Diluted wine intoxicates quickly because the watery constituent takes it quickly into the blood.

The wise person will avoid drinking wine when fasting or before the limbs have been refreshed in warm water, or after vigorous exercise; for both these entail a strain on the brain and nerves, and render a person liable to develop cramps and amentia; they produce either actual illness or at least undue heat.

Frequent intoxication breaks down the constitution of the liver and brain, weakens the nerves and tends to produce diseases of the nervous system, apoplexy, and sudden death.

When wine is taken to excess it is changed, in the case of some persons, into a bad kind of bilious humour or, in the case of others, into pure vinegar. In both cases, the changes in the stomach are very injurious.

Some persons claim that it is an advantage to become intoxicated once or twice a month, for, they say, it allays the animal passions, inclines to repose, provokes the urine and sweat, and gets rid of effete matters.

The most detrimental of the effects of wine is that upon the brain. That is why those who are not strong in that way should take but the very least amount of wine, and diluted.

If called to a person who has drunk wine to excess, emesis should be procured as speedily as possible. Failing that he may drink a considerable quantity of water, with or without honey. When emesis has been procured, he should bathe in a full length bath. Then he should be thoroughly rubbed with oil, and left to go to sleep.

To give wine to youths is like adding fire to a fire already prepared with matchwood. Young adults should take it in moderation. But elderly persons may take as much as they can tolerate.

Wine is borne better in a cold country than in a hot one.

If a person wishes deliberately to take his fill of wine, he must take no food, or anything sweet. The [Persian] white broth [made of meat, onions, butter, cheese, etc.] may be allowed; also grated bread steeped in broth made with fat meat cut into pieces. He should have an inunction. He should avoid physical labor or exercise. Then after the meal, when he wishes to drink, he should accompany it with almonds, salted lentils and a condiment prepared with salted capers.

It is an advantage to include in the menu cabbage boiled with meat; olives boiled in water, and the like. For this conduces to drinking more wine. Anything which lightens the fumes of the wine is also helpful for instance the seeds of Syrian beet; cumin, dry rue, pennyroyal, Nabathean salt, cardamoms; and more particularly, any aliments which are viscous and glutinous, for they aggregate the fumes (i.e., oily, sweet and viscous articles of food) and prevent inebriety in spite of drinking so much wine, by restraining the rapidity with which the wine enters the blood.

Inebriation is rapid: (1) when there is weakness of the brain; (2) when there is an abundance of humours; (3) when the wine is strong; (4) when the food is scanty; (5) when the regimen is itself depraved; and (6) when the wine is taken continuously (for a long time).

When the cause of the ready inebriation is weakness of the brain, the remedy is to use the epithemes named in the chapter on catarrh, give sedatives, and avoid fluids.

The following syrup averts inebriety: one part of juice of white cabbage; one part of juice of unripe pomegranate, a half-part of vinegar. Simmer. Take one ounce before taking the wine. The following is another remedy: pills containing salt, rue, black cumin. Eat pill by pill. The following is another: take seeds of Syrian beet, cumin, peeled bitter almond, pennyroyal, absinthe, Nabathean salt, cardamom, dry rue.

A person who is not afraid of a hot mixture may take two drachms by weight in a draught with cold water, fasting.

For agents which restore from inebriety, let the person take water and vinegar several times one after the other, or whey water and junket. Let him sniff at camphor and sandalwood. Put cold repercussives over his head, such as rose oil and wine vinegar.

The treatment of inebriety is discussed in Volume III.

1.10. Concerning Sleep and Wakefulness

If it is desirable to get a person unconscious quickly, without his being harmed, add sweet smelling moss to the wine, or lignum aloes.

If it is desirable to procure a deeply unconscious state, so as to enable the pain to be borne which is involved in painful applications to a member, place darnel water into the wine; or administer fumitory, opium, hyoscyamus (half-drachm dose of each); nutmeg, crude aloeswood (4 grains of each). Add this to the wine, and take as much as is necessary for the purpose. Or, boil black hyoscyamus in water, with mandragore bark, until it becomes red. Add this to the wine.

The causes of natural sleep and of lethargy; their opposite states (the waking state, and insomnia); their effects; the remedial measures applicable when they are baneful; the significance of each; and all other points about them, have been dealt with in brief in the appropriate place. The special treatment will be discussed later.

Physiological effects of sleep—at present we may say that sleep in moderation: (1) assists the vegetative drives in their functions; (2) brings the sensitive drives into repose and in so doing (3) renews and restores them and thereby (4) arrests the dissipation of the breath (the vital power). Hence, the digestion of the food in the several stages we have named is accomplished. Sleep also remedies the weakness due to the dispersal of the breath (vital power) in various ways; namely, by bodily fatigue, by coitus, by anger or violent emotional disturbance, and the rest.

Furthermore, a moderated amount of sleep brings about an equilibrium in regard to quantity and quality of the humours, and therefore it has a humectant and warming action, which is specially advantageous for the aged, who need their moisture preserving and renewing. That is why Galen said: "Every night I partake of a little packet of herbs and lettuce combined with aromatics; the former because they induce sleep, the latter because they rectify the coldness of the lettuce." And he said: "I am now careful to obtain sleep because I am an old man, and the humidity which sleep brings is beneficial to me."

This then is the way to obtain sleep. And if a bath be taken after the digestion of the meal has been completed, and plenty of hot water is poured over the head, this will be an additional help. A still more efficient method will be mentioned under medicaments.

Conditions to observe regarding sleep—healthy persons should pay attention to the subject of sleep: it must be moderate, properly timed, and excess must be avoided. And on the other hand they must avoid the injury resulting to mental and all other faculties from remaining awake too long.

However a person is often driven to keep awake, and refrain from sleep owing to a dread of syncope and loss of strength. The best sleep is that which is deep; and that which occurs after the food has passed on from the upper part of the intestine, and after the flatulencies and eructations which may have followed have subsided; for to sleep on this is detrimental in many ways, though the person himself may not know it; it keeps him turning from side to side in his sleep; it hinders digestion; and it does injury. For this reason, if the passage of the food out of the stomach is delayed, he should take a walk for a little while, and then retire to sleep.

It is also bad to go to sleep on an empty stomach, as this is weakening. It is bad to go to sleep after repletion, before the food has left the stomach, because sleep cannot be deep under such circumstances, and the sleeper will keep turning from one side to the other all the time. For when the natural drives are busy with the work of digestion at a time when it is accustomed to be asleep, the fact of being prevented from waking up is disturbing to the natural drives; so they become dulled and the process of digestion is disorganized

It is also bad to go to sleep during the day, for in this case illnesses depending on humidity and catarrhal states are brought about; the color of health passes off, the spleen becomes heavy, the nerves lose their tone; lack of vim and a poor appetite are noticed, and inflammatory conditions and fevers often appear.

Among the reasons for the injurious effects are: liability to sudden interruption of sleep whereby the natural drives become dulled.

Among the good qualities of sleeping by night are that it should be continuous and deep. If a person is accustomed to sleep during the day, he should not suddenly discard this custom but do so gradually.

Posture in sleep—the best way to sleep is to begin on the right side, and then turn round to the left. If one begins by lying face downward, it greatly helps the food to digest, because by this posture the innate heat is conserved and magnified.

It is a bad practice to sleep on the back. It courts the development of grave maladies like apoplexy, paralysis, and nightmare, because the effete matters then tend to accumulate in the tissues of the back, where they are held and prevented from entering the natural channels which are in front, such as the nostrils and palate. Persons who are accustomed to sleep on their backs often become debilitated, for their muscles and members become weakened; also because one side cannot alternate with the other, seeing that such persons quickly return to the supine position, the back being more powerful than the sides. The consequence is that such persons sleep with their mouth open, for the muscles which keep the jaws closed are too weak to maintain them in that position. (A special chapter is given on this subject in the special part).

1.11. Matters Which Are Best Described Later

We leave over until later the discussion of coitus and its constitution, and the measures to be taken to correct errors in this function, though strictly they belong to this place. It is discussed in the special part.

At this point also, one would discuss the agents for procuring evacuation of the bowel, and how to deal with any antagonistic influences towards them. We reserve this subject to the section dealing with treatment and the chapter on purgatives. However, we may say here that a person who wishes to maintain his health should procure evacuations by the bowel, the urine, the sweat, and the sputum.

We shall also explain how one may assist and regulate the menstrual flow of women, in order that you may become familiar with this.

1.12. Strengthening, Fattening and Enlarging Weak Organs

Members (limbs) which are weakly and undersized may be strengthened and caused to grow and develop during the period of growth, up to the final limit for growth, by the use of a suitable degree of massage and of a suitable form of exercise, steadily persisted in. Also by the use of pitch plaster. An exercise consisting of holding the breath [according to proper rules] is also effective, especially for the respiratory organs (thorax, lungs).

For instance, let us suppose the legs to be underdeveloped; the person takes a short running exercise; then a certain amount of massage is given; then a plaster of pitch is applied. Next day the running exercise is prolonged a little, but the amount of massage remains the same as on the first day. On the third day, the massage given is to the same extent as before, but the exercise is still further lengthened, taking care to stop short of distension of the vessels, for this would show matters are lodging in them which might be antecedent to some inflammatory process or repletion specifically met with in them: varices, and elephantiasis being an instance of such. Therefore, should there be any suspicion of anything of that nature, shorten the exercise to the original degree, reduce the massage; enjoin rest in the recumbent position; raise the affected member. Thus, if the persons have a wasted (lit. dried up) leg, raise it by the foot, and apply massage from its distal towards its proximal end.

To carry this method out for parts related to the organs of respiration the thorax, for example we proceed to apply a bandage to the lower parts, making it moderately tight, and of uniform breadth. Then we instruct the patient to exercise his arms, and to breathe as deeply as possible, uttering a loud sound the while (this may be assumed to a singing exercise, a sustained note being produced for as long as possible at each breath), light massage being applied as well. (This subject will be fully discussed in the Special Part on Beauty Culture, God willing).

1.13. The Types of Fatigue Affecting Exercise Management

There are three kinds of lassitude, and we may add a fourth. There are two modes. The three varieties are: the ulcerose (painful), the tensive (cramp-like), and the inflammative (congestive). The fourth variety which we add is the chapped, dry, and thin.

1.13.1. Painful Fatigue

Painful fatigue or ulcerose lassitude is a form in which the subject experiences the sensation of ulcers upon the body or in the depths of the skin. The deeper the sensation the greater is the lassitude. The sensation may be evoked by contact with the skin; or it may be evoked by movement. Sometimes it gives rise to the sensation of pricking with needles, with a dread of movement, and the subject lies extended because of the weakness of his shoulders and arm-pits. If the degree of lassitude is still greater, there is a goose-skin. When it is still greater, tremors and fever appear.

1.13.2 Cramp-like Fatigue

The cause of this kind of lassitude consists in an abundance of tenuous and pungent effete matters, a liquefaction of the flesh and fat in consequence of the over-vigorous exercise, and, lastly, the presence of depraved humours in the vessels, which results in changes in the blood, whereby it loses its healthy character; these abnormal products pass into the skin and affect it. This form of lassitude is the lesser evil which such substances produce. If they should become mobile, goose-skin will result. If they move about still more actively, tremors result. Sometimes the pungent humours detach themselves from the others, leaving the crude humours in the vessels. Sometimes the crude humours are situated in the flesh.

With cramp-like fatigue there is the sensation of the body being broken, of heat, of tension or being in a stretched condition, and has a dread of moving himself or straightening his back from the bent position. This is specially the case when the condition follows physical labor. This condition arises from the retention of waste matters in the muscles which are otherwise in themselves normal; it is not due to acridity or gaseous matters in them. The fibers are separated from one another, and there is a state of lightness or heaviness. This is often the result of want of sleep.

When not associated with want of sleep, the case is different and more serious. Here the muscle fibers are stretched lengthways.

1.13.3. Congestive Fatigue

With congestive or inflammative fatigue, the body is hotter than usual. The part is as if distended, being swollen, and of corresponding color. Distress is felt when the part is touched, or when the patient tries to move, for this brings out the tension or stretching which is like the sensation in an inflamed or bruised tissue: Aeg.]. The deep-seated pain is called ostealgia. The cause is abundance of waste matters in the muscles.

1.13.4. Dry Fatigue

This is a state wherein one feels a sensation of being dried up in an unusual degree. It follows (a) undue exercise, the chyme being normal; (b) twisting the body back sharply; (c) sometimes it is owing to dryness of atmosphere; (d) deficient nutrition; (e) fasting too much. [There is great disinclination for any movement: Aeg.].

1.13.5. Complex Fatigue

The two modes of lassitude. (a) That following exercise; this is less serious. It is rectified by suitable measures. (b) Spontaneous; this is a forerunner of illness. Special measures must be used for its cure.

These two forms or modes may be combined, the matters which give rise to each being present together, both those which arise spontaneously, and those which result from exercise.

The regimen for the simple form is known to you. That for the compound form entails the following rules: in the first place pay most attention to avoid the danger of the condition by dealing with the underlying cause. There may be three sources of danger: severity, the nobility (of the organ), and the substance involved. If two, or three are concurrent, the condition is more serious unless the one of them which outstays the other is more potent and therefore overrules them. For instance, inflammative lassitude is more severe, and the ulcerose form is nobler; but if the substance underlying the ulcerose is far from equilibrium and from the natural course, it forms a restraining influence over the two modes of the inflammative lassitude, by virtue of this nobility and strength, and takes precedence over it. But if the relation be not so very remote, the inflammative lassitude would take the precedence.

1.14. Stretching and Yawning

Stretching comes on when effete substances have accumulated in the muscles. For this reason the desire to stretch oneself is often experienced after sleep.

If these humours become superabundant they give rise to goose-flesh and trembling and shivering. If they increase to a still greater degree, fever develops.

Yawning is really a form of stretching, when this takes place in the muscles of the jaws, lips and chest. Should it arise without any apparent reason in a person seemingly healthy, and not at an appropriate time, and to an unusual degree, it is bad. In such a case, it is best when it comes on at the end of digestion, because then it is due to the effete substances being expelled.

Stretching and yawning may be due to external cold, to thickening of texture of the skin, whereby exit of certain humours becomes restricted; to being awakened from sleep before it has finished; to postponing the evacuations.

1.15. The Treatment of Fatigue After Exercise

Moderately diluted wine is good for this condition, provided there is no contra-indication.

1.15.1. Painful Fatigue

We may say that the chief object to be attained in treating lassitude is to prevent it from being followed by many diseases, including fevers. Ulcerose lassitude is dealt with by reducing the amount of exercise if that be the cause. If at the same time there is an over abundance of humours, they need to be expelled. If there be a transient sensation of nausea and satiety these effects are counteracted by fasting, evacuation through the bowels, and dispersal of the humours in the subcutaneous tissues by the use of plenty of light massage, carried out with oil devoid of astringency. Exercise is then resumed. On the first day the nourishment should consist of the usual quality of foods, in lessened amount. On the second day the diet should consist of humectants. If the vessels be patent, and there be crude serous humour in the mesentery, friction may help to mature it, especially if one could bring the virtue of calefacient medicines (digestives) to bear on it. Very good (calefacients) are: willow oil, oil. anethi; oil of chamomile; and the like. A decoction of beet roots in oil, prepared in a double-vessel; ointment of mallow roots; oil of the roots of cucumber asininus and of bryony; oil of sweet-scented moss; and any oil in which the latter (moss) has been incorporated. [Galen recommends discutients and restorative exercise.]

1.15.2. Cramp like Fatigue

In regard to cramp like or tensive lassitude, the object in view in treating this is to relax the indurated tissues by means of a little gentle massage with oil heated in the sun; tepid baths in which the patient stays a considerable time; or, better, to take the bath once or twice a day, followed each time by an inunction; complete rest. If it becomes necessary to procure an abstersion of the vessels, or if the oil of the inunction has become dried up, repeat the inunction and administer moist foods in only small amount. It is more important that the amount should be small in this case than in that of ulcerose lassitude. Exercise is sufficient to disperse this kind of lassitude, and cleanse out [the substances which cause it].

If tensive lassitude have arisen simply by the presence of gross superfluites, these must be evacuated. If it has arisen from flatulencies, it is dispersed by the use of such as cumin, caraway, and anise.

1.15.3. Congestive Fatigue

In regard to congestive fatigue or inflammatory lassitude. There are three aims in treatment of this condition: to relax the tense parts, to cool the heated parts, and to remove the superfluities. These are achieved by the use of plenty of tepid oil, by vigorous light massage, by a prolonged stay in a bath of tepid water (on the warm side), and by sufficient repose [and by repeated inunction: Aeg.].

1.15.4. Dry Fatigue

With dry fatigue or arefactive lassitude, the first day: the normal regimen for maintaining health is to be continued, save that the bath water should be hotter, because very hot water has a contracting effect upon the skin. This action is not as detrimental as that of cold water, for in this case there is a risk of the cold penetrating into the body, already dry. The cause of the wasting (wrinkling, shriveling of the skin) may also lie in the fact that the skin is usually relaxed.

The second day of the restorative treatment consists in the use of gentle restorative exercise of a light character. The bath should be carried out in the same way as on the first day and the patient should then plunge into cold water, to make the skin shrivel, and to reduce perspiration to a minimum. In this way the skin keeps moist. For water will come in contact with the body as soon as there is sufficient heat in it to counteract the dryness of the skin. And these two factors mutually assist one another in combating the injurious effect of the cold. The injurious effect is greater if the person comes quickly out of the water into which he has plunged.

1.16. General Principles

Those affected with lassitude need wholesome food, which must contain little moisture, and should be taken at the end of the first morning hour. Friction may be given on a later occasion, towards evening. The supper must then be taken later still.

The removal of superfluities from the body must also be procured, using massage with sweet, or willow oil [cf. the modern oil. betula oil, or oil of wintergreen]. The abdominal muscles are not touched unless lassitude is present in them. In that case, give light inunction and increase the amount of such food as is not too heating.

One should take care that exercise should stop short of producing any sign of lassitude. Then proceed to reversion exercise in order to draw matters towards the skin by the moderate amount of movement. Having reached the skin, massage during the time of resting between the exercises will finally disperse these substances.

As regards bathing, person's condition is the guide. If the bath should induce tremor, the last degree of lassitude has been reached. How much more is this true if fever comes on after the bath. In such a case the bathing must be stopped, and recourse must be had to evacuation [of various kinds] and the rectification of the temperament. As long as the water is moderately hot, and the bathing produces none of these adverse symptoms, one knows that it is beneficial to bathe.

If there were non-matured humours in the vessels, the first measure to take would be to apply whatever was suitable for the lassitude, and the next would be to endeavor to make the crude humours mature and become attenuated, and then to expel them. If they were plentiful, order rest; forbid exercise, because rest is the great digestive. Avoid bleeding because by this means both pure and crude matters are expelled.

It is injurious to procure purgation before maturation. There is no harm in inducing dieresis. But avoid drugs which are very heating, for otherwise the crude humour would be caused to diffuse throughout the body, and facilitate its action.

Diet: include pepper, capers, ginger, vinegar of capers, vinegar of garlic, vinegar of spurge, and dried dates, and the well-known confections (i.e. of quince, apples, prunes, etc.), according to measure. The appearance of a sediment in the urine informs us that maturation has occurred. One may now order wine to complete the maturation and to procure dieresis. The wine must be delicate and clear, and must not excite vomiting.

1.17. The Management of the Side Effects of Exercise

1.17.1. Physical Conditions Which Follow Exercise

We may first speak about the states, and then pass on to the subject of the regimen applicable for lassitude of autogenous origin.

1.17.2. Flabbiness

Rarefaction of the skin: very often this is the result of insufficient massage, and of bathing. The treatment consists in dry massage, tending slightly to rough, using an astringent oil for the purpose.

1.17.3. Hardness

Thickening of the skin (induration, constriction, tightness, tenseness, shriveling, sclerosis, corrugation may be the result of: (a) cold; (b) an astringent bath; (c) over-abundance of effete matters, (d) thickening and aggregation of coarse particles of effete matters; (e) change in the effete matters [or immatured humours] in the direction of viscidity in consequence of which they cannot pass through the pores of the skin, and so block them; (f) exercise, for this draws the humours out from the deeper (or remote) tissues, if no other cause for this has previously been in operation; we (g) residence in a dusty place; and (h) too rough and vigorous massage.

When it is due to cold and astringency, the color of the skin is pale [because it is stretched hard and tight], and the bodily warmth returns only slowly; sweating is delayed. The skin becomes red again on resuming exercise. Such cases should be treated thus: the stay in the cold room of the bath must be very short, and the water must not be very cold; then go into very hot water; turn the patient from side to side, then on to the belly, then on to the back. The slab on which he lies the while must be of medium heat. Do this until perspiration sets in. Then anoint with thin [sweet: Aeg.] oils of a hot and resolvent character [oil of dill, of black poplar: Aeg.].

Cases due to exercise are distinguished by the absence of the above-named sign. The skin is discolored by sweat and sordities. Such cases are treated by getting rid of such superfluities as may be present, and then carrying out a bath and inunction regimen of resolvent character.

Cases due to exposure to fine dust, or due to the use of too much rough massage, are much more in need of the bath than of inunction with oils. Soft massage is to be employed both before and after the bath.

1.17.4. Excessive Moisture

Rarefaction of the skin may be associated with weakness (asthenia). This may be the result of (a) excessive exercise, especially if subsequent massage were insufficient; (b) overindulgence in coitus; (c) too frequently repeated baths. The treatment of such cases therefore consists in the use of restorative exercises, and of dry massage, for which an astringent oil is used in order to obtain a hardening effect. The diet should include humectants in small amount, which are moderately calefacient or moderately infrigidant or slightly inclined to be hot.

1.17.5. Excessive Dryness

The same sort of treatment is used for asthenia, wakefulness, sadness, dryness in the nerves (or the state which follows on anger). In such cases, if the patient finds the digestive process of the food is depraved, the reversion exercises are not good; indeed no exercises are to be recommended.

When the cause of the weakness is an over indulgence in baths, in eating and drinking, and inactivity, the patient suffers from undue humidity in the tissues (especially the tongue), and the activity of the limbs is impaired. Should this depend on some antecedent cause, the special treatment for that will become necessary.

In the case of any other causes which we have named—wine, undue inactivity, undue moistening effect of the bath—the best thing to do is to anoint the body, use vigorous exercise, employ rough dry friction without oil, or a massage with the aid of a small amount of a calefacient oil.

When a person experiences undue dryness of the skin of the hands, this belongs to the category of arefactive lassitude. The treatment is the same as for that condition.

1.18. The Treatment of Spontaneous Fatigue

The ulcerose state is recognized when the humour upon which it depends is within or without the vessels. The humour is shown to be within the vessels by: (1) the urine being fetid; (2) the nature of the previous diet, for some articles of diet give rise to an undue proportion of superfluous matters in the blood; some articles of diet give rise to too few superfluous matters; or these matters are expelled too speedily, or medicinal treatment may become necessary for them; and (3) the character of the fluids taken if wine, whether clear or thick.

From all such data one comes to the conclusion that the site is within the vessels; if it is not found, the condition is extravascular.

In cases where the lassitude from superfluities is of extrinsic origin, and the vessels are unobstructed, it is sufficient to carry out reversion (restorative) exercises, and follow the regimen, to an increased degree, which we have indicated for cases of ulcerose lassitude due to exercise. But if the case belongs to the other group, one should not order exercise, but inactivity, sleep, fasting. Then, towards each evening, the abdomen should be anointed with oil, followed by a bath in moderately hot water, if his condition is such that he will stand the bath.

The diet should be of the character already stated: one which makes good chyme, fluid or semi-fluid [lit. able to be sucked, e.g. through a tube or spout], not viscid, and not particularly nutritious. Examples of such foods are: barley, frumenty, game (provided it is delicate), syrupus acetous with honey, mead, light white wine. A wine which is matured and diuretic need not be forbidden, but to begin with one would prefer to administer a wine which is slightly sour or rather yellow. Afterwards one changes to a white and light wine.

If this regimen proves ineffective it will show that the excess of humour present needs evacuation. Should it be the sanguineous humour, do a venesection [or scarify the ankles: Aeg.]. Otherwise, procure purgation, making your choice between them according to the proportion of sanguineous humour which you judge to exist. But take care not to do either if the vitality is low.

To ascertain the kind of humour concerned, one considers the character of the urine and sweat; and the tendency towards sleep or wakefulness. It is a bad sign if sleep is banished in spite of a good regimen.

If one has ascertained that there is a deficiency of good blood in the body, and that the immature acrid humours are in excess, one must not bleed the patient or purge [or let him bathe (Aeg.)], but procure complete rest. Order attenuant foods and fluids; avoid any fluid nourishment which is calefacient, but choose such as has a sharp or biting or incisive quality: e.g. syrupus acetous, with honey [acid wines, capers with vinegar and honey: Aeg.]. If it be necessary to increase the power of the attenuants, put a little pepper into the food, and into the barley-water [especially as there is generally hypogastric flatulence: Aeg.]. Cumin and pepper may be needed to counteract the immaturity of the humours (i.e. acrid matters which have not been properly digested) administering them either before or after a meal, or at bedtime, according as seems best to you. The dose is a small tablespoonful. Pennyroyal is not so good, for it is overheating.

Now if one is absolutely certain that the immature humours are not it the vessels but in the tissues (lit. roots of the members) one orders massage; laxative oils, especially in the mornings; heating drinks—whose heat passes to the skin; a long rest; then a moderately hot bath. Prescribe pennyroyal fearlessly, whilst being sure to give it before meals and exercise.

If it be necessary to aid the gastric digestion before a meal, do not give a strongly penetrative remedy like pennyroyal, but choose cumin and pepper in small dose. Quince may also be used. One could administer more of the latter, if one decides that the extraneous heat of the body would not be much greater in degree by giving it. Beneficial remedies: inunction with oil of chamomile, of aniseed, of sweet marjoram, etc.-whether given alone or combined in wax. Their action is increased by resin, alone or with twice its volume of its oil.

When one has ascertained that the immature humours are in the vessels, and at the same time outside them, one would become more anxious. Do not lessen your efforts in consequence. If there be as much within as without, first aim at procuring the maturation of the humour; pepper may be used for this purpose. To that, if one wishes, one may add parsley, and an equal weight of anise. In this way a greater degree of dieresis will be procured. Or, if one so desire, one may admix with it a little pennyroyal, and at the same time lessen the amount of cumin and pepper. These are lessened step by step until at last there remains simply nothing but pure pennyroyal. As soon as the (foreign matter) in the vessels has become digested, and has passed on out of them, one has to deal with that which is exterior to them. Pennyroyal will be useful for this purpose, whereas it was impeditive at first. Where the two conditions occur concurrently one must take special care not to attract the impure matter forcibly towards the surface of the body, or to the interior organs either. Therefore, one should not risk producing emesis too soon, or purging before the humours are rendered tenuous, and have been cut and matured. Exercise is also not ordered.

When the lassitude has passed away, and the color of the skin is more healthy, and the urine normal (mature), plenty of massage is given and exercise in small amount. One considers whether there is any chance of a relapse, for in that case one would pause in these measures. If it appears that a relapse will not occur, the customary life with regard to bathing, inunction, massage, exercise, is gradually resumed. Finally the strength of the ointments used is brought back to the customary.

If a relapse is threatening, with a sensation like that of ulcerose lassitude, the regimen must be taken up again. If the relapse threatens without that sensation of ulcerose lassitude, the treatment is by reversion-exercise.

If the signs are ambiguous, and the sensation of lassitude is not marked, order rest.

The cause of pensive lassitude is repletion without depravity of the humour. If the temperament is unhealthy, order venesection and an attenuant regimen. In the type of person of which we speak, the treatment is by attenuants and a certain amount of incisives; after that one helps the cure by using appropriate agents.

Treat inflammative lassitude by venesection. The choice of vein depends on the part most affected with lassitude or the part in which the condition began; if it be the head, use the cephalic vein; if the chest or back, use thee basilic vein; if the other members are chiefly affected, or there is no distinction of priority, bleed from the median vein of the arm. It may be necessary to bleed on the second or even the third day On the first day, one bleeds as soon as the lassitude appears, otherwise the condition may become established. The proper time to bleed on the second or third day is sunset.

On the first day, the diet should consist of barley water alone, or juice of frumenty as long as there is no fever. If there is fever, give barley water alone. On the second day give a cooling or attempered oil like almond oil. On the third day give a salad made with lettuce or cucumber (or, members of the gourd family), or garden mallow [or, beet, Aeg. or sorrel in cold broth: Aeg.], and give rock fish in white broth (i.e. a special dish or recipe) and forbid drinking [cold: Aeg.] water as much as possible during this day.

If by the third day, the patient feels nausea, or, if he has an appetite but the stomach cannot digest the food, let him have mead, or a light white wine, or an attempered white wine. After the evacuations, take care not to give a great deal of food all at once, for undigested food will be drawn into the blood. This is due to three factors: (i) when there is not much food, the stomach greedily holds it, and its retentive power—is antagonistic to the attractive power of the liver. When food is plentiful, the stomach is not greedy of it, and then its expulsive power helps the attractive power of the liver. The same holds good with each receptacle in turn in regard to that which comes next into play; (ii) when there is much in the stomach, it does not get digested as well; (iii) the presence of plenty of food means that there will be much nutriment for the blood, and the vessels [greedily absorb the chyle before it is digested: (Aeg.) and they themselves are incapable of digesting it.

1.19. Concerning the Bodies of Those with Abnormal Temperaments

The temperament (constitution) of the body may be defective either from some deleterious influence, or from the natural course of events beginning from birth. In the former case the temperament was appropriate for a certain length of time, until persistent faulty regimen has produced a change which itself remains persistent. In the latter case the defective constitution has been present from the outset (of conception).

In the first group of cases, the error is in quantity or in quality, and the nature of the case is revealed by a study of the form of the body. The remedy is to have recourse to the corresponding contrary.

The second group of cases shows a depravity of the state of the body in that there is a change either in the original constitution or in the course of advancing years of life.

We therefore begin the subject by going into the regimen of the elderly.

Endnotes
Introduction by Laleh Bakhtiar

1 Seyyed Hossein Nasr, *Three Muslim Sages*, pp. 23-24.
2 The Islamic medical tradition is the part of reference of this great textbook of Avicenna (Ibn Sina) which served to heal millions of people as this was the only medical textbook for 700 years in Europe alone. Translated into Latin, it served as the basis for Shakespere's psychology, among others. St. Thomas Aquinas has said: Anything Avicenna says is correct.
3 Nader Ardalan and Laleh Bakhtiar, *The Sense of Unity*, p. 11.
4 Ibid., p. 11.
5 Ibid., p. 13.
6 Ibid.,p. 13.
7 Ibid., p. 19.
8. R. A. Nicholson, *Rumi, Mystic and Poet*, p. 31.
9. Nader Ardalan and Laleh Bakhtiar, *op. cit.*, p. 19.
10 *Ibid.*, p. 19 which quotes S. H. Nasr, *Three Muslim Sages*, p. 112.
11 Seyyed Hossein Nasr, *Islamic Science: An Illustrated Study*, p. 161.
12 According to the Ayurvedic system, there are three bio-energies called *dosha (arkan)*. They are *vatha* [nervous spirit]: driving force. It relates mainly to the nervous system and the body's energy; *pitta* [animal spirit, fire] relates to digestion, metabolism, enzymes, acid and bile; *kapha* [natural spirit] relates to mucous membranes, phlegm, moisture, fat and lymphatics.

Seyyed Hossein Nasr points out: "It is worth drawing attention to the similarity between the words *ruh* and *rih* (the wind or air) in Arabic and to the Galenic doctrine that through the air breathed by the organism the life-force enters the body. It is also of significance to note that in Arabic as in many other languages the words for breath (*nafas*) and soul (*nafs*) are related. Therein lies a profound cosmological principle which is also related to the invocation of the Name of God (*dhikr*) as the central technique of Sufism for spiritual realization." *Sufi Essays*, p.27.

13 Seyyed Hossein Nasr, *Science and Civilization in Islam*, pp. 223-224.
14 Called *prana* or energy of life in the Ayurvedic system, it is comprised of energy which changes according to our circumstances, our diet, our lifestyles and the world around us. Some are positive and some are negative. We have to live in a way to attain energy balance. Energy controls the functions of every cell, thought, emotion, and action.

O. Cameron Gruner's Remarks

1 This was actually Gruner's conclusion, but because it explains the content of The Canon so well and because today we have grown so distant from Avicenna's concepts, we have placed it before Gruner's original introduction, which follows and expounds the differences between Avicenna and "modern medicine."
2 Altounyan, Lancet, 1928, ii, 684.
3 St. Thomas Aquinas, *Summa Theologica*, p. 177.
4 See Introduction by O. Cameron Gruner, Doctrine of "the Constitution"
5 See notes to Avicenna *on Psychology*, Details Regarding the Emotions.
6 See Avicenna *on Diagnosis Signs and Symptoms*, Details Regarding Odor.
7 See Avicenna *on The Temperaments*, Details Regarding Age.
8 Notes to Avicenna *On the Four Temperaments*, Application of the Doctrine; notes to Avicenna *on Psychology*, Details Concerning Some of the Drives; List of Terms Applicable to Mental Faculties.
9 Notes to *On His Psychology*, List of Terms Applicable to Mental Faculties.
10 St. Thomas Aquinas, *Summa Theologica*, p. 203.
11 See Avicenna *on the Breath*.
12 For other cycles see Avicenna *on Illness*.
13 See Introduction by O. Cameron Gruner, Doctrine of "the Constitution."
14 Notes to Change in Vibration-rate.
15 Vallery-Radot, *Precis de Pathologie Medicale*.
16 *Uruj* (ascent), *nasul* (descent), *jalal* (majesty), *jamal* (beauty), *qada* (fate), *qadr* (destiny).
17 Cf. Bechold 112, Sckade 137, Pearson and Wyllie 160 and many other authorities.
18 See *On the Diagnosis of Signs and Symptoms*.
19 See *On the Diagnosis of The Pulse*.
20 See *On the Diagnosis of Signs and Symptoms*.
21 See *On Medicine and its Topics*.
22 Many other points are noted in Part Two.
23 See *On Treating Diseases, Disorders, Obstructions, Swellings and Managing Pain*.
24 M. O. Stanton, *An Encyclopedia of Face and Form Reading*.
25 Sir A. Garrod, *The Huxley Lecture on Diathesis*.
26 See *On the Classification of Types of Disease*.
[Footnotes 37-51 not featured]
52 See *On Medicine and its Topics*.
53 See *On Medicine and its Topics*.
54 See *On Medicine and its Topics*.
55 *Ibid*.
56 See *On Medicine and its Topics*.
57 J. P. Bruce, *Chu Hsi: Philosophy of Human Nature*, p. 168.
58 Chuang Tzu, Giles translation, p. 170.
59 *Ayurveda*, 1924, i, I.; and see also Weber, *History of Indian Literature*.
60 Forke, *Chinesische Mystik*, pp. 242, 243.
61 Lancet, 1927.
62 Cf. Forke, *ibid*.
63 Hume quoted by Maher, *Psychology*, p. 238.
64 Kempis, *Imitatio Christi*, ii, II.

65 St. Thomas, *Summa Contra Gentiles*, i, 53.
66 *Gulshan-i raz*, couplet 299, p. 30.
67 *Essays in Zen Buddhism*, p. 185.
68 *Ibid.*, p. 200.
69 *Ibid.* p. 306.
70 *Rose Garden*, 1st ed., p. 120.
71 J. P. Bruce, *Chu Hsi: Philosophy of Human Nature*, i., 182.
72 The real authorship of the Libellus on the power of the hearts is disputed. Arnold of Villanova translated it into Latin (ca. 1235-1312).
73 Huineng, Susuki, *Essays in Zen Buddhism*, p. 203.
74 *Ibid.*, p. 223.
75 *Kempis, Imitatio Christi*, i., 5.
76 St. Thomas Aquinas, *Summa Theologica*, Dominican translation.
77 Ibid., liv; lv. 2; lviii. 3,4; vol. 3, p. 51-87; Pegues, *Catechism of the Summa Theologica of St. Thomas Aquinas*, p. 18.
78 F. Hartmann, *The Life of Paracelsus*, p. 217.
79 Ed. Hughes, *Lancet*.
80 Sauvage, *Catholic Encyclopedia*, xii., 313.
81 Mercier, *Manuel of Modern Scholastic Philosophy*; Logique, 1904; de Wulf, *Catholic Encyclopedia*, xii., p. 26.
82 Maher, *Psychology*, p. 520.
83 Cf. Maher, *Psychology*, pp. 35, 36; and especially Wundt, *Catholic Encyclopedia*, xii., p. 35.
84 Maher, *Psychology*, p. 9.
85 In. Met. I., lect. 2.
86 *Summa Theologica*, II-III, q. 45, art. i.e.
87 *Ibid.*, ad. 2.
88 *Ibid.*, q. 9, a. 2, ad 3.
89 St. Thomas Aquinas, *Summa Contra Gentiles*.
90 *Ibid.*, ii. 3, I. p. 5.
91 *Catechism of the Council of Trent*, 1545-1563.
[Footnotes 92-123 not featured]
124 *Arabian Medicine*, p. 34.
125 *Die Augenheilkunde des Ibn Sina*.
126 *Arabian Medicine and Its Influence on the Middle Ages*, p. 139.
127 E. G. Browne, *ibid.*, p. 26, 27.
128 *Manuel of Modern Scholastic Philosophy*.
129 Maher, *Psychology*, endnote, p. 31.
130 J. B. Bruce, *Chu Hsi and His Masters*, p. 137.

On Healthy Living: Exercising, Massaging, Bathing, Eating, Drinking, Sleeping and Treating Fatigue

1 Rumi says:

How happy is he who takes advantage of early days and pays his debt to God.
Those days when he has power, health, energy of heart and strength.
That state of youth, like a verdant and fresh garden, yielding produce and fruit unstintingly.
The springs of strength and eager desire flowing and the soil of the body verdant through them (*Mathnawi*, p. 107).

The real object of conserving the energies of the body likes in the attainment of spiritual development. The actual bodily occupation is itself, if we will it so, the practical means of that attainment. The energy of will to associate this means of worship with the subjugation of the vices inherent in our frailty must be employed during the early years if we are not to find ourselves in old age powerless to advance along the critical stages of the journey to the only true goal. This principle underlies the idea of "right regimen."

The soil of the body and the desires having been consistently tilled and purified and tended, the coming of old age cannot but also reveal spiritual blossoms full of delight for others. Do not then wait, says Rumi till:

The soil becomes barren, dry and poor.
Never do fine plants grow from barren soil.
When the water of energy and the water of eager desire cease,
He derives no benefit from himself or from others;
The eyebrows hanging over like a crupper-strap;
The eyes watery and dim;
The face through old age like the back of a lizard;
The articulation and taste defective and the teeth useless;
The day late, the ass lame, and the road long;
The workshop (i. e., the physical body) gone to ruin.
And the work disorganized,
The roots of a bad nature fixed firmly in him,
And the power to tear them up diminished (*Mathnawi*, p. 107-8).

A picture admirable of the state of affairs in old age and also full of significance in regard to the well-being of the soul.

2 The value of exercise: (1) it hardens the organs and renders them fit for their functions; (2) it results in a better absorption of food, aids assimilation, and, by increasing the innate heat, improves nutrition; (3) it clears the pores of the skin; (4) it removes effete substances through the lungs; (5) it strengthens the physique.

Vigorous exercise invigorates the muscular and nervous system.

3 Equitation "strengthens the body especially the stomach more than any other mode of exercise. It clears the organs of special sense and renders them more acute. But it is most inimical to the chest" (Antyllus). The mental excitement of hunting is good for many diseases.

"Dancing," said Hippocrates, "is beneficial for amenorrhea and has been used for procuring abortion. Swimming in the sea has a warming effect and strengthens the body and renders it thin. It is beneficial for dropsy, skin-eruptions, elephantiasis. But it may be injurious for the head for the head and nerves. The body must be rubbed with oil first" (Oribasius).

4 Reading aloud in a high tone helps to remove redundant humours through the skin. Reading in a moderate tone helps the insensible perspiration throughout the body, attenuates effete matters, and gets rid of saliva, mucus and phlegm by coughing. Frigid people should read aloud frequently because of its warming effect. This method of exercise requires control and judicious management if the system is full of depraved humours or if the stomach is loaded with crudities, because otherwise noxious gaseous substances are distributed all over the body. Ritual: first empty the bowels then anoint the body, then sponge the face and lower parts with water. The tone of the voice should be moderate at first, and the person should walk about while speaking. Then a louder tone should be used and verses should be repeated several times.

5 The urinary signs of the proper time for undertaking exercise are specified in Aegineta. The urine should be deep yellow, because this shows that the digestion has long since been completed. If the urine is moderately pale, it shows that the digestion has only just been completed. An evacuation of the bowels is here indicated. If the urine be watery, it shows that there is still some undigested chyme in the stomach.

6 Two kinds of leprosy are distinguished by the Arabs: *baras* and *juzam*. The former is "white" and the latter is "black." The latter is leprosy of the joints. Both are ascribed to dietetic errors, especially fish-eating and milk drinking (Burton, iii. 370). The term used in the present passage is *juzam*.

7 Polenta=*sawiq*=ptisane (Lane). This is native frumenty and green grain (mostly barley), toasted, powdered, mixed with dates or sugar, and eaten on journeys when cooking is impracticable. It is carried in a meal-sac (Burton, iv. 491).

8 Soured milk is milk artificially soured. It is eaten with rice and is a component of salatah, cucumber salad (Burton, *iv.* 132; who adds, "All nomads who live on milk never take it fresh."

9 *Kabab*: this is mutton or lamb cut into small squares and grilled on skewers. It is the equivalent of our roast meat (Burton, iv. 154).

10 Strictly speaking, instructions on diet to the patient should rest upon practical acquaintance with the culinary art as having a prior place over the questions of forbidding and allowing such and such articles of food, food values, and the like. The form in which a given article in the dietary is to be given is of real importance, and the combinations into which the foods enter require notice at least to the same extent as is done with the ingredients of a medicinal prescription. Mutual decompositions occur with foodstuffs either before or after ingestion. Interactions may render the " composite " indigestible, or non-palatable, or actually harmful; the use of too little of one ingredient in a recipe or of too much should be prevented; the temperature to which the mixture is exposed—the rate at which that temperature is reached, whether too quickly or too slowly-whether it is maintained steadily or whether through some mismanagement the "mixture" was allowed to cool noticeably in the midst of the operations—all such details call for consideration both as to a possible explanation of persistent gastro-intestinal trouble, and as to guiding the management of any ailment in any system or organ.

The displacement of *materia medica* from its ancient throne is partly to be ascribed to a cessation of attention to detailed knowledge about herbs and the part which horticultural skill and care, as well as climatic conditions and geographical factors play in the production of efficacious remedies; it is also ascribable to entirely insufficient attention to the preparation of the recipes-for these originally were exacting as to manner of compounding; and both these types of indifference rest upon a skepticism as to the possibility of such details being of the least importance. In the absence of knowledge on these points, the decriers of the use of drugs, and of complex prescriptions speak unjustifiably.

So, again, in the matter of the preparation of the invalid's food, or the dietary for the chronic ailment, it is reasonable to plead for that care whose real importance is every day proved by those who, having the means, will desire their meals from some one chef in preference to another.

In the whole of the preceding chapter, Avicenna is referring to a cuisine which is foreign to us. Perhaps of all European countries, Spain offers the nearest approach to his. Those who have been in the East, and have inquired into the practical details in their cookery recipes, not merely such as may be available in written form, but also such as are actually carried out in well-to-do establishments or by the humbler housewife, (for in this country also there is much difference between Beeton and actual practice) are more easily able to follow Avicenna's nomenclature.

Very little research suffices to convince the enquirer of the very great scope of this subject. Interesting as it is, it would, therefore, lead too far to attempt proper discussion in these pages. It must suffice to insist that the names of foods and dishes which Avicenna gives bear a different meaning to those same names with which we are familiar. Confusion would only be prevented by giving the names in the original language. Many of the words are Persian; some of the dishes are Syrian; others are Indian.

The following notes from Lane and Burton will serve to show the type of dishes which may be regarded as characteristically Arabian.

"Among the more common dishes are the following: lamb or mutton cut into small pieces, and stewed with various vegetables, and sometimes with peaches, apricots, or jujubes, and sugar; cucumbers or small gourds, or the fruit of the black or white eggplant, stuffed with rice and minced meat, etc.; vine-leaves or pieces of lettuce-leaf or cabbage-leaf, enclosing a similar composition; small morsels of lamb or mutton roasted on skewers, called kabab. Fowls simply roasted or boiled, or boned, and stuffed with raisins, pistachio nuts, crumbled bread, and parsley; and various kinds of pastry and other sweets.

"The repast is frequently commenced with soup, and is generally ended with boiled rice, mixed with a little butter, and seasoned with salt and pepper; or, after this, is served a water-melon or other fruit, or a bowl of a sweet drink composed of water with raisins, and sometimes other kinds of fruit, boiled in it, and then sugar, and with a little rose-water added to it when cool. The meat, having generally little fat, is cooked with clarified butter, and is so thoroughly done that it is easily divided with the fingers. A whole lamb, stuffed in the same manner as the fowls above mentioned, is not a very uncommon dish. (Lane, 159 *Nights*, i. 171.)

"They brought him . . . dishes of poultry besides other birds and brewises, fritters and cooling marinades." (*Night* 415, Burton). . . . "a mess of cooked pomegranate seed." (*Night*, 712.)

"A very common kind of pastry is a pancake, which is made very thin, and folded over several times like a napkin; it is saturated with butter, and generally sweetened with honey or sugar; as is also another kind which somewhat resembles vermicelli." (Lane.)

- *adasiyah*: soup of yellow lentils, made by boiling them in water till nearly dissolved, and then adding vinegar, coriander, and salt.
- *faturat*: junket: a light food for early breakfast, of which the fatirah-cake was a favorite item. (Burton, *vi*. 160.)
- Fruits: almond, almond-apricot apple, apricot, banana, bergamot pears bitter orange, blood-orange, cherry, citron, date, fig, grape, hazelnut, jujube, lemon, lime, lote, mulberry, olive, peach, plum, pomegranate, quince, shaddock, sugar-cane, sweet-orange, sycamore-fig, walnut, water-melon. (Lane, *i*. 30I; Burton, *v*. 28I-287)
- *hisrimiyah*: a broth of kid's flesh, lamb, and fowl seasoned with *hisrim*, the juice expressed-from the grape while unripe.
- *jamar*: palm-pith eaten with sugar (Burton, *v*. 284).
- *kaak al-id*: "cake"; bun; a special sweet cake eaten with dates and sherbets. (Burton, *iv*. 394.)
- *kabab* .
- *kunafah*: vermicelli cake; a favorite dish of wheaten flour worked somewhat finer than our vermicelli, fried with *samn* (butter melted and clarified) and sweetened with honey or sugar. It may be-sweetened with bees' honey (*Night* 989) in preference to.the frequently used various syrups. (Burton, *vi*. I50.)
- *sawiq*: polenta.
- *sikbaj*: acid minced fresh meat, dressed with vinegar and honey, or with acid syrup. Raisins, a few figs and chiches were sometimes added. (Lane, *i*. 435.)
- *shurayk*: a cake or bun, the size of the palm of the hand, with two long cuts and sundry oblique cross cuts, made of leavened dough, glazed with egg and clarified butter, and flavored with spices (cinnamon, curcuma, artesmisia, prunus mahalab, and sundry aromatic seeds specified by Lane as aniseed, nigella, absinthium (Artemisia arborescens) and camphor, etc. (*Nights*, v. 509.)
- Soured milk.
- *yakhmi*: stew. A complicated broth prepared from rice and meat. (Burton, iv. 387.)
- *zardah*: a rice dish. Rice dressed with honey and saffron (*ib*. p. 385).
- *zirba*j: a sour meat dish similar to sikbaj (above).

Notes

Notes

CPSIA information can be obtained
at www.ICGtesting.com
Printed in the USA
FSHW010807140220
67021FS

9 781567 447934